CU00926898

A TEXTBOOK FOR DENTAL SURGERY ASSISTANTS

A TEXTBOOK FOR DENTAL SURGERY ASSISTANTS

S. F. PARKIN MDS (Lond), FDŞRCS (Eng)
*Senior Lecturer in Children's Dentistry, The Dental School of the
 School of Medicine, University College, London
Honorary Consultant, University College Hospital Dental
 Hospital, London.*

JANET R. OAKELEY
*Registered Dental Surgery Assistant
City and Guilds' Technical Teacher's Certificate
Formerly tutor to the dental surgery assistants at University College
 Hospital Dental Hospital, London*

faber and faber
LONDON · BOSTON

First published 1973
by Faber and Faber Limited
3 Queen Square, London WC1N 3AU
Revised reprint 1977
Reprinted 1980
Second edition 1983
Revised reprint 1986
Set by Goodfellow & Egan Ltd, Cambridge
Printed in Great Britain by
Redwood Burn Ltd, Trowbridge, Wiltshire
All rights reserved

British Library Cataloguing in Publication Data

Parkin, S.F.
    A textbook for dental surgery assistants.—2nd ed.
    1. Dentistry   2. Dental assistants
    I. Title   II. Oakeley, Janet R.
    617.6RK60.5

ISBN 0–571–18070–1

Contents

Preface to the Second Edition

This book is intended for Dental Surgery Assistants at all stages of their career, but it should be of particular interest to those in training. We have aimed to provide a basic account of the theory and practice of the various branches of dentistry for use during the initial period of learning basic skills and gaining experience at the chairside, and also as an aid to revision. In selecting the material included we have paid close attention to the course of study suggested by the British Examining Board for Dental Surgery Assistants in preparation for the National Examination.

This second edition has been extensively revised to include much new material and additional illustrations. Changes in terminology, materials, drugs and techniques are constantly occurring in modern dentistry as research continues to increase the scope of our knowledge and practice. Where possible we have tried to indicate the specific areas in which these changes are taking place: as we say 'the trained Dental Surgery Assistant owes it to herself and her profession to keep alert and up to date'.

We wish to acknowledge our profound debt to all those from whom we have learnt and to those whose work and research over the years have advanced modern dentistry to its present stage.

We are most grateful to the many friends and colleagues who have read sections of our manuscript and have helped us by giving valuable constructive criticism. So many people have assisted us in this way that we cannot begin to name them all here.

We thank our artists, Mrs Audrey Besterman, Ashley S. Lupin and John M. Perkins for providing us with such excellent illustrations and for their meticulous attention to detail. We also thank Mrs K. Holden, tutor to Dental Surgery Assistants and Mr Charles Day, chief photographer, University College London Dental School for additional photographs of DSAs carrying out procedures.

We are also indebted to the Amalgamated Dental Co Ltd for their generous permission to reproduce numerous illustrations of instruments from their catalogues. The dental charts on page 93 are reproduced by kind permission of the Board of Governors of University College Hospital.

We are particularly grateful to the Examining Board for Dental Surgery Assistants for permission to reproduce a selection of examination questions from recent papers.

We are most grateful to Miss P. A. Downie, Medical and Nursing Editor, Faber and Faber, whose cheerful encouragement and painstaking care have contributed so much to this edition.

Finally, we again give our special thanks to our families without whose patience, tolerance and support we would not have found the time or endurance to write this book at all.

S.F.P. and J.R.O.
1983

THE DENTAL PROFESSION

Dentistry, in one form or another, has been practised throughout history, for toothache has always been one of the worst discomforts of mankind. Treatment was crude and of limited extent until medical science began to supplant ignorance.

For many centuries dentistry in Europe was mainly confined to the extraction of teeth until, in the 18th century, men like the French dentist Pierre Fauchard (1678–1761), author of the authoritative book *The Surgeon Dentist*, and John Hunter (1728–1793), in London, began to lay the foundations of modern dentistry.

Thus the dental surgeon replaced the ancient tooth drawer and dental science and practice developed rapidly. Dentistry became a discipline requiring its own course of study when the Medical Act of 1858 was passed, and the Royal College of Surgeons of England instituted an examination and diploma in dental surgery. Soon the established universities began to offer degrees in dental surgery.

The Dentists' Act 1921
With more people becoming dentists Parliament passed the Dentists' Act of 1921 which made it illegal for unregistered persons to practise dentistry. The General Dental Council only accepted names for the Dentists' Register of those practitioners who fulfilled certain stringent qualifications regarding training. Thus the practice of dentistry was controlled, and high standards of professional education and conduct among dentists were promoted.

The evolution of the Dental Surgery Assistant (DSA)
Chairside assistants were of various standards throughout Britain until the Association of British Dental Surgery Assistants was founded in 1940 with the objects of protecting and furthering the interests of those assisting dental surgeons. An examination was introduced in 1947 and there are now

11

training programmes available at all major dental hospitals. The status of the DSA is continually being raised and there is a growing awareness in the dental profession that the use of the trained chairside assistant is an essential part of dental practice. She is no longer a 'housekeeper' but a member of the dental team, serving dentistry in many ways – on the telephone, at the chairside, in the laboratory, in the office, meeting new patients, educating the patient, dealing with radiographs and, on her dental surgeon's behalf, the DSA is a goodwill ambassadress at all times. The procedures that a DSA may perform are determined by the British Dental Association's guidelines; in practice the duties of the DSA will depend on her particular qualifications, experience and the specific needs of her employer. The Association of British Dental Surgery Assistants aims to improve the training and career opportunities of its members and to gain the best advantage and benefits from qualification. In 1964 a voluntary National Register of Dental Surgery Assistants was established, compiled by a joint committee of representatives from the British Dental Association and the Association of British Dental Surgery Assistants, listing all those who have passed an approved examination.

THE MODERN DENTAL PROFESSION

The governing bodies of the dental profession are the General Dental Council, the examining bodies (Universities and Royal Colleges) and the Department of Health and Social Security which is responsible for the National Health Service.

The General Dental Council (GDC) ensures the standards of dental training and practice. Only those whose names appear on the dental register are permitted to practice. Once registered, any misdemeanour, e.g. unprofessional conduct such as: (a) covering (associating with an unqualified person who is practising dentistry); (b) abusing the drug regulations; (c) abusing professional relationships; (d) falsifying certification of documents; and (e) advertising or canvassing for patients, may be disciplined by striking the practitioner's name from the Register. As far as the GDC regulations are concerned, a DSA counts as a non-registered person who is therefore forbidden to carry out dental treatment for patients apart from her normal duties of assisting a registered dentist at the chairside.

The educational and examining bodies such as the Royal Colleges and the Universities, monitored by the GDC to maintain standards, provide a series of examinations for registrable degrees for which undergraduate students study for up to five years at recognised schools.

The National Health Service (NHS) Act of 1946 which became operational on 5th July 1948, introduced a free health service into the

United Kingdom for the first time. Today, the NHS is involved with most of the dental practice in Great Britain. It controls, monitors and finances dental practice carried out in general practice, hospital and community services. It demands certain specific obligations from the practitioner who is willing to undertake this work and sets the fees for items of service which may be paid directly from the NHS and partially from contributions by the individual patient at the time of treatment. (The dental surgeon is forbidden to carry out treatment both under the NHS and privately for a particular patient during one course of treatment.) It also requires prior permission before certain extensive courses of treatment are provided.

The NHS is managed from the Department of Health and Social Security (DHSS) on behalf of the Minister of Health and the lines of communication, which vary from time to time because of reorganisation, pass through the district health authority (DHA) to the district dental officer (DDO) who is in charge of the local community services, the family practitioner committee (FPC) in charge of general dental practice, and the dental estimates board (DEB) which deals with the monthly payments for completed courses of treatment and is also concerned with granting prior approval for certain types of treatment.

From time to time a sample of cases of completed treatment are called in for examination by another dental surgeon, employed by the DHSS, whose job is to ensure that the standards of treatment under the NHS are being maintained at all times. The DHSS dental officer may also examine patients if there is a problem about agreeing payment for unusual items of treatment. Up-to-date booklets providing detailed guidance with regard to NHS dental treatment, forms and documents are sent to all NHS practitioners from time to time and the DSA student should read one.

The British Dental Association (BDA) is a professional body which most qualified dental surgeons voluntarily join and which is alert to protect the interests of dental surgeons. Thus it is involved in negotiations on the profession's behalf with the government and other bodies and provides a network of professional groups throughout the United Kingdom which meet regularly for lectures, discussions and conferences. It publishes the *British Dental Journal* and maintains a professional library, reading room and museum at its headquarters in London where trained staff are available to advise members on all aspects of dentistry.

Dental practice can be carried out in a variety of circumstances, for example the commonest place is in general dental practice where the dental surgeon may be treating his patients under the rules of the NHS or by private arrangement with the individual patient. There are also occasions when domiciliary visits are necessary and the surgeon and assistant attend the patient in his own home.

The hospital services are provided by the NHS and here the dental surgeons hold a similar status to that of their medical and surgical colleagues, i.e. consultants with their registrars and house surgeons. Patients may be referred to such specialised hospital dental units when they present special problems of diagnosis and treatment – for example major oral surgery, road traffic accidents, advanced orthodontic treatment and other specialties. University dental staff follow training similar to that of members of the hospital dental service and clinical teaching staff usually hold honorary contracts in the NHS which give the staffs parallel status. However, considerable importance is also attached to their teaching and research abilities, and published work.

The community services are also part of the NHS. Here the dental surgeon is a member of the salaried staff controlled by the district dental officer, whose surgery, staff and materials are provided for him. He is primarily responsible for treating children in local schools, but in addition cares for pre-school children, expectant and nursing mothers and the handicapped patients in his community. He is also concerned with preventive care and dental health education for the community. Operative work is generally carried out in permanent clinics, but in some areas the dentist may work in a specially equipped mobile clinic.

Some practices may be associated with industry, for example within the environs of a large factory complex or a large multiple department store, so that the employees lose the minimum of time having treatment, and their dental welfare is ensured.

Within the armed forces dental surgeons join as commissioned officers and provide dental care for servicemen and their families.

Dental team

The dental team, working together to provide dental care for their patients as efficiently as possible, is always headed by the dental surgeon with his DSA, and in addition may also include the receptionist, other DSAs, the dental hygienist, the dental technician, and, in the community services, the dental health educator and the dental therapist.

Dental surgery assistants are employed in all areas of dentistry and have duties which are both varied and interesting, but their chief task is to assist the dentist and the patient before, during and after treatment. In the community dental service and in smaller general practices the duties of a DSA may well include the work of a receptionist (admitting patients, filing, making appointments, and handling general correspondence). In larger general practices where a receptionist is employed, the work of the DSA will be more concerned with helping the dental surgeon at the chairside in the provision of treatment.

Dental receptionists, although not directly concerned with the provision of dental treatment, contribute greatly to the smooth running of the practice which is of direct benefit to the patient. The dental receptionist is the first person patients see when they come to the surgery, or hear when they telephone, so tact, sympathy, a pleasant manner with an ability to put patients at their ease are all requirements of her work. She is also responsible for filing patients' notes, case histories and other paperwork necessary in dentistry – arranging appointments, sending out reminders, communicating with the NHS authorities and so on. Although there is no formal training, clerical and secretarial skills are obviously desirable.

Dental technicians are highly skilled craftsmen following four or five years' training, who construct dentures, crowns, bridges and orthodontic appliances according to the dental surgeon's requirements. They are important members of the dental team but do not provide treatment direct to members of the public. Many work in the general practice field but there are possibilities for specialisation (e.g. maxillo-facial work, where the technician works in conjunction with a consultant oral surgeon to help restore the patient's face and oral structures after radical surgery, or following accident or deformity).

Dental hygienists, although not employed in all practices, have an important part to play in the dental team taking some of the dentist's workload. A hygienist who has completed a training course and passed the examination for the Certificate of Proficiency in Dental Hygiene is then entitled to entry in the Roll of Dental Hygienists and only those thus enrolled are permitted to practise under the direction of a dental surgeon. Duties include the scaling, cleaning and polishing of teeth, the application of preventive materials, such as fluoride and fissure sealants, to the teeth and instructing patients in the care of their mouths to keep teeth and gums healthy. With the demand for places to train as a hygienist so great, most schools expect applicants to have trained first as a DSA who may also have taken the Royal Society of Health's Diploma in Dental Health Education.

Dental health educationalists will have taken the Royal Society of Health's Diploma in Dental Health Education, and are employed in some cases to instruct patients and other members of the general public.

Dental therapists, after completing a two-year course, are allowed to work only in the community service or hospital and may carry out simple dental treatment for children under the direction of a dental surgeon who will examine the children first and prescribe written treatment plans within certain defined limits. The dental therapist may scale and polish teeth, apply fluoride and fissure sealants, provide simple fillings and extract deciduous teeth under local infiltration anaesthesia, and conduct dental health education. She may often be helped in the surgery by a DSA.

Doctors may visit the practice as anaesthetists, and become members of the team to administer the necessary general anaesthetics for patients.

15

Other important visitors to the practice will include the representatives from dental companies and the engineers called in to repair and service existing dental equipment.

Chapter One

ANATOMY AND PHYSIOLOGY

Anatomy. This is the study of the form and structure of the body and of the relationships of its constituent parts to one another.

Physiology. This is the study of the function of the normal body as a whole and of its component parts and organs.

The cell. This is the microscopic unit from which all living organisms are built. Cells are composed of material called *protoplasm* which contains a watery solution (water = 70 per cent of the total cell volume) of proteins and small amounts of fats, carbohydrates, vitamins and salts.

Basically, an animal cell is a highly organised structure made up of a *nucleus* surrounded by a quantity of *cytoplasm* which is contained within the boundaries of a flexible *cell membrane*. The cell membrane is a permeable wall which allows selected materials to move in and out of the cell. The cytoplasm is concerned with the metabolism of the cell. The nucleus controls all cell processes and plays a vital part in cell division for it contains the *chromosomes* which carry hereditary information. Although microscopically no two types of cells are identical, there is a common pattern of organisation and generalisations can be made.

Cells are active, living units and demonstrate the basic characteristics of all living things: they use oxygen, they take in food for energy, growth and repair, they excrete waste products, at some stage they grow, they can reproduce (by cell division), they respond to outside stimuli and they can be killed.

TISSUES

In the human body the cells have *differentiated* into various types, each specialised to serve a particular purpose. This specialisation means that cells are no longer capable of a separate existence but depend in turn on other groups of cells to collect oxygen and food and bring nutrition to them.

Tissues are made up of large numbers of identical cells which have developed to carry out a special function. They fall into four main groups.

Epithelial tissues. These serve as protective layers and membranes covering the surfaces of the body inside and out. For example, they form the skin and line the respiratory, digestive and urinary tracts. A secretory type of epithelium is found in *secretory glands* such as the salivary glands, the sweat glands and the tear glands.

Muscular tissues. These have the power of contraction. Three types are found in the body: *voluntary* or *striped*, e.g. the muscles of the limbs and the muscles of mastication; *involuntary*, *smooth* or *unstriped*, e.g. the muscles of the gut; and *cardiac*, the special muscle of the heart walls.

Connective tissues. These bind, connect and support the body and form a framework for the organs. *Areolar* tissue is a loose packing material. *Adipose* tissue contains fat. *Fibrous* tissue forms tendons and ligaments. *Bone*, the hardest connective tissue, forms the skeleton. *Cartilage* or gristle is found in various forms and hardnesses, e.g. on the surfaces of joints, in the flexible external ear, in the intervertebral discs of the spine.

Nervous tissues. Nerve cells and their long processes form the brain, spinal cord and the nerves passing to all parts of the body. *Motor* or *efferent nerves* conduct (transmit) impulses from the brain and spinal cord to motivate all action in the tissues, e.g. a muscle contraction. *Sensory* or *afferent nerves* conduct impulses to the brain from peripheral receptors, e.g. the touch or thermal receptors in the skin. Many main nerve trunks are *mixed* and contain both sorts of nerve fibres.

An organ. This is any differentiated part of the body devoted to a special function, e.g. tongue, eye, tooth, heart, lung or kidney.

ANATOMICAL TERMS

In anatomy the human body is studied and described as if it were standing in an upright position with the head erect and the eyes looking forward. An imaginary *median plane* runs vertically through the centre of the head, neck and trunk dividing them into left and right halves. The relative distances of structures from the median plane are described by the terms *medial* (nearer to) and *lateral* (further from). *Anterior* lies to the front or *ventral* side of the body and *posterior* to the back or *dorsal* side, while *superior* and *inferior* are used to indicate high and low positions. *Internal* and *external* describe the relative distances of a structure from the centre of a body cavity. *Superficial*

18

and *deep* indicate the relative depths of structures from the surface of the body.

Systematic anatomy

For study purposes it is convenient to consider the different combinations of tissues, organs and structures according to the functions they perform.

1. The locomotor system: the skeleton, joints and muscles.
2. The circulatory system: the heart, blood vessels and blood.
3. The respiratory system: the air passages and lungs.
4. The digestive system: the gastro-intestinal tract and its associated organs.
5. The nervous system: the brain and peripheral nerves including the special senses.
6. The urogenital system: the urinary and reproductive systems.
7. The endocrine glands: the ductless glands which secrete hormones.

(This chapter includes only those sections of the general systems that are of importance to the dental surgery assistant's studies.)

LOCOMOTOR SYSTEM

Skeleton

This is the bony framework of the body, supporting the soft tissues and protecting the vital organs within the skull, vertebral canal, rib cage and pelvis. Many bones can move as levers about the joints in response to the action of attached muscles. The skeleton forms about 15 per cent of the total body-weight.

Bone is a living tissue able to respond slowly to external influences, e.g. prolonged stress, by the remodelling action of bone-forming cells, *osteoblasts*, and bone-dissolving cells, *osteoclasts*. It acts as a storehouse of available calcium for the body.

Each bone is served by nutrient blood vessels and is also covered by a highly vascular tissue called the *periosteum*. The outer layer of a bone is very hard and dense, the *compact bone* or *cortex*, while the deeper internal layers are composed of lighter, spongy bone, the *cancellous bone*. Many bones have a central cavity, the *medullary cavity*, e.g. within the shaft of a long bone of a limb, containing the fatty *bone marrow* which is the site of formation of red and white blood cells. The medullary cavity also serves to make the bone lighter.

The axial skeleton. This is made up of the skull, hyoid bone, vertebral column, ribs and sternum.

The appendicular skeleton. This is formed of the bones of the upper and

19

lower limbs and the limb girdles (pelvis, collar-bones and shoulder-blades).

SKULL

This is made up of the eight bones of the *cranium* (the 'brain box') and the 14 bones of the *facial skeleton*.

Cranial bones (Fig. 1/1)

One *frontal* bone which forms the forehead and the upper margins of the eye sockets (the orbital cavities).

Two *parietal* bones which together form the roof and side walls of the cranium.

One *occipital* bone which forms the back and part of the floor of the cranium (the base of the skull). This bone is perforated by a large opening, the *foramen magnum* (foramen: an opening or hole, especially in bone) through which the lower part of the hind brain passes to join the spinal cord. On the external surface, on either side of this opening are the bony facets, the *occipital condyles*, which support the skull at the top of the spinal column.

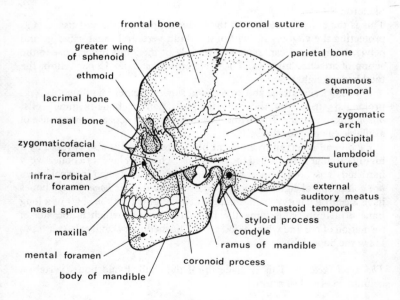

Fig. 1/1 Lateral aspect of the skull

Two *temporal* bones which form the lower side walls of the cranium. They contain the middle and inner parts of the hearing apparatus and also provide the fixed base for the *temporomandibular joint*.

One *sphenoid* bone which forms part of the floor of the cranium.

One *ethmoid* bone which lies at the front of the cranium forming the roof of the nasal cavity between the two orbits and is perforated by numerous holes (foramina) through which pass the *olfactory nerves* for the special sense of smell.

Facial skeleton (Figs. 1/2 and 1/3, and Chapter 2)

Two *nasal* bones which form the bridge of the nose.

Two *zygomatic* bones, the cheek or malar bones which join the zygomatic processes of the temporal bones to form the *zygomatic arches*.

The *maxilla* which is formed of two halves and thus consists of two bones. It forms the lower border of the orbits, the sides of the nose aperture and also the upper jaw.

One *mandible* which forms the lower movable jaw and supports the teeth.

Two *palatine* bones which form part of the roof of the mouth.

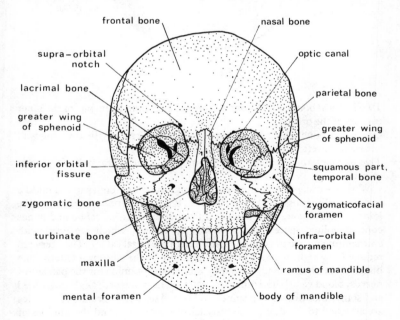

Fig. 1/2 Frontal aspect of the skull

21

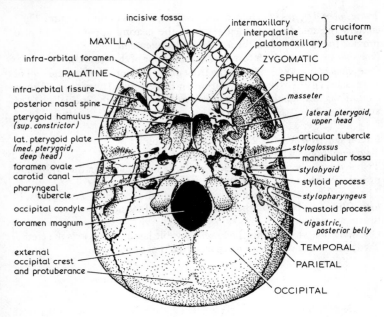

incisive fossa

intermaxillary ⎫
interpalatine ⎬ cruciform
palatomaxillary ⎭ suture

MAXILLA

infra-orbital foramen

PALATINE

ZYGOMATIC

SPHENOID

infra-orbital fissure

posterior nasal spine

pterygoid hamulus
(sup. constrictor)

masseter

lateral pterygoid,
upper head

lat. pterygoid plate
(med. pterygoid,
deep head)

articular tubercle

styloglossus

mandibular fossa

foramen ovale

carotid canal

stylohyoid

styloid process

pharyngeal
tubercle

stylopharyngeus

occipital condyle

mastoid process

foramen magnum

digastric,
posterior belly

external
occipital crest
and protuberance

TEMPORAL

PARIETAL

OCCIPITAL

Fig. 1/3 Basal aspect of the skull

Two *lacrimal* bones which contain the tear ducts and form part of the inner corners of the orbits.

One *vomer* bone which forms part of the nasal septum (the dividing wall between the left and right halves of the nasal cavity).

Two *inferior turbinate* bones which form part of the lateral wall of the nasal cavity.

With the exception of the mandible and some tiny bones in the middle ear (the auditory ossicles) all the bones of the skull are united by immovable joints called *sutures*. The maxillary, frontal, ethmoid and sphenoid bones contain hollow spaces, the *paranasal air sinuses*, which are lined with epithelium and are in communication with the nasal cavity. They serve to reduce the weight of the bony skull and also act as voice resonators. The bones of the skull are perforated by numerous foramina for the passage of nerves, blood vessels and other structures. The bones are rough and ridged and sometimes drawn into spines and processes where groups of muscles are attached to them, e.g. the muscles of mastication and the muscles of facial expression.

Spine

This is also called the back-bone or vertebral column and is a flexible column made up of 33 bones called *vertebrae*. There are 7 *cervical* in the neck; the second cervical (axis) has the odontoid peg around which the atlas, or first cervical vertebra, moves when the head is rotated or in nodding. There are 12 *thoracic* associated with the ribs, 5 *lumbar* in the loins and, fused into two immovable groups, 5 *sacral* and 4 *coccygeal* vertebrae (the sacrum and the coccyx) which form the back of the pelvic girdle. The movable vertebrae are separated by intervertebral discs of fibro-cartilage. Down the *vertebral canal* formed by the column of vertebrae and their processes runs the spinal cord from the brain giving off 31 pairs of spinal nerves which pass out through the intervertebral spaces.

Ribs

There are 12 pairs of ribs: 7 'true' ribs extending from the vertebral column to the *sternum* (breast bone), 3 'false' ribs attached with cartilage to the sternum and 2 'floating' ribs which are unattached in front. Together they form the *rib cage*.

Joints

These occur at the union of any two or more bones of the skeleton. They may be freely movable, e.g. the limbs, slightly movable, e.g. the vertebrae, or fixed, e.g. the skull or sacrum.

In movable joints the articulating bone surfaces are covered in smooth cartilage and the joint is contained within a fibrous capsule (the joint cavity) and held together by firm ligaments. The inside of the joint cavity is lined with a *synovial membrane* which secretes a lubricating fluid. Movable joints are subclassified by the mode of action, e.g. hinge, ball and socket, sliding and pivot joints.

Skeletal muscles

These are the contractile groups of striped muscle which cause bodily movement under the voluntary control of the nervous system. They are usually attached at each end: the *origin* is the end which remains stationary when the muscle contracts while the *insertion* attachment is drawn towards it. Muscle attachments may be to bone, cartilage, ligaments or skin. Strong movements require large muscles or groups of muscles working together. Muscles tend to work in opposition to other groups of muscles and by a fine balance of contraction and relaxation between them, delicate, controlled movements can be made. Muscles are generally described according to their shape, position, direction of movement or function.

23

CIRCULATORY SYSTEM

This system comprises the heart, blood vessels and the lymphatics.

Heart (Fig. 1/4)

This is a hollow muscular pump which provides the motive power for the passage of blood to the tissues. It lies in the centre and slightly to the left of the mid-line of the chest. It is divided into left and right sides by the *septum*, each side being further divided into two chambers, the upper *atrium* and the lower, thicker-walled, *ventricle*. The atria communicate with the ventricles through openings guarded by valves; on the right side the three-valved *tricuspid valve* and on the left the two-valved *mitral valve*. The right ventricle pumps blood to the lungs through the semilunar *pulmonary valve* while the left ventricle pumps blood to the rest of the body via the *aortic valve*. (On average the heart pumps 70ml of blood 70 times a minute for 70 years.)

Arteries carry blood away from the heart to the tissues. *Veins* carry blood toward the heart from the tissues (see also pages 28 and 211). *Capillaries* are very fine blood vessels in the tissues which link the arteries and the veins and through their walls allow nourishment, oxygen, waste products, and so

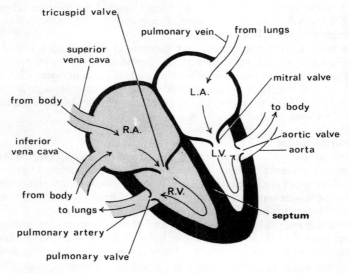

Fig. 1/4 The heart. The right atrium and the right ventricle are shaded to indicate that the blood they contain has not been oxygenated

on to be interchanged between the blood and the tissue fluid. *Lymphatics* are small vessels which act as a drainage system to carry away some of the fluid (lymph) which has exuded from the capillaries and, filtering it through the lymphatic glands, return it to the blood vessels in the thorax. They play an important part during inflammation.

CIRCULATION OF THE BLOOD (Fig. 1/5)

Systemic circulation

Blood is pumped from the left ventricle of the heart into the *aorta*. In turn the aorta splits into smaller arteries and these subdivide further to serve all parts of the body. (The first branches from the aorta, the *coronary* arteries, serve the heart muscle itself.) The walls of the arteries are muscular and this helps to maintain the *blood pressure*. The pumping action of the heart causes pulsations in the arterial blood and this pulse can be felt in superficial arteries such as those in the wrist. After passage through terminal *arterioles*

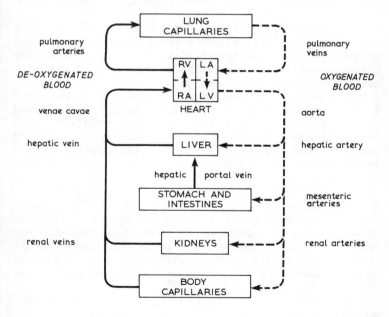

Fig. 1/5 The circulation of the blood (diagrammatic).

into the capillaries, the blood flows back to the heart through the veins which empty through the *venae cavae* into the right atrium.

Pulmonary circulation

The returned systemic blood is pumped from the right atrium through to the right ventricle and thence out through the pulmonary artery to the lungs and into the pulmonary capillaries for gaseous exchange of oxygen and carbon dioxide. The oxygenated blood is returned to the left atrium via the pulmonary veins and is pumped through the left ventricle again.

Portal circulation

Blood from the stomach and gut, containing nutrient materials, is collected in the portal vein and transported directly to the liver. In addition the liver also has its own hepatic artery from the systemic circulation.

Blood

This is a 'fluid tissue' made up of liquid blood plasma and its contained cells, a total of about five litres in an adult. Blood cells are of different types:

Red cells (erythrocytes). There are 3.9 to 6.5×10^{12}/litre of blood. These cells are very elastic and can accommodate themselves to the shape and dimensions of the narrowest vessels of the blood vascular system. They contain a protein complex, *haemoglobin*, concerned with the transport of oxygen. *Anaemia* means lack of haemoglobin.

Plasma contains substances which cause foreign red cells to stick together (agglutinate) and great care has to be taken if blood is transferred from one patient to another (transfusion) to make sure that they both belong to compatible *blood groups*. (Broadly, the groups are 'A', 'B', 'AB' and 'O'. 'A' plasma agglutinates 'B' cells, 'B' plasma agglutinates 'A'. 'AB' plasma, 'the universal recipient', has no agglutinins and 'O', 'the universal donor', has both.)

White cells (leucocytes). These amount to 5.0 to 10.0×10^9/litre. Granulocytes and polymorphonuclear leucocytes form 70 per cent of the total leucocytes. They are subdivided into neutrophils, eosinophils and basophils according to their staining reactions. The 'polymorphs' are mobile cells which deal with infection and invading bacteria and remove injured or dead tissue cells, usually by engulfing and digesting the undesirable material.

Lymphocytes form 25 per cent of the total white cells and take part in the defence mechanism and increase in numbers in chronic infection.

Monocytes form five per cent of the total white cells and may also play a part in the defence against chronic infection.

Platelets (thrombocytes). There are 2.5 to 3.5×10^{11}/litre. They have an important role in blood coagulation – the haemostatic mechanism.

Plasma. This is concerned with the transport of the blood cells and itself contains many dissolved materials including fibrinogen, the protein concerned with coagulation, and *antibodies* which provide immunity to specific organisms or toxins.

Coagulation. When blood is shed from a vessel, it sets into a jelly (blood clot) within five minutes (the clotting time). This jelly is formed by a complex chemical action between factors in the platelets and in the plasma whereby countless microscopic threads of *fibrin* are formed which entangle the cells. The jelly contracts and the defibrinated *serum* (a clear yellowish fluid) is exuded. This coagulation mechanism renders the circulation system 'self-sealing' following injury to a blood vessel and is the first stage in repair.

Functions of blood
1. The transport of oxygen to the tissues.
2. The transport of nutrients to the tissues.
3. The transport of waste materials and carbon dioxide from the tissues.
4. Assistance in the defence mechanism against infection and injury.
5. The transport of chemicals and hormones to the tissues.
6. Assistance in the distribution of heat throughout the body, and temperature control.
7. Coagulation and sealing of injuries to the circulatory system.

RESPIRATORY SYSTEM (Fig. 1/6)

Oxygen is required for most of the chemical reactions in the body and in the production of heat and energy, carbon dioxide being produced as a waste product. *Respiration* means taking in oxygen and passing out carbon dioxide. The respiratory system is composed of the lungs, air passages and the mechanisms for expanding and contracting the walls of the thoracic cavity to *inspire* (draw in) and *expire* (breathe out) the air. During inspiration, air (which contains about 21 per cent oxygen) is drawn in through the *nose* where it is warmed and moistened before passing on through the *nasopharynx* and the *larynx*, between the vocal cords, down the *trachea* (windpipe, held open by rings of cartilage), through the smaller branching *bronchi* and via the small terminal *bronchioles* into the *alveoli* (air sacs) of the lungs. Once here the air is brought into close contact with a rich network of blood capillaries. The haemoglobin of the red cells, having a great affinity for oxygen, is converted to *oxyhaemoglobin* and carried back

27

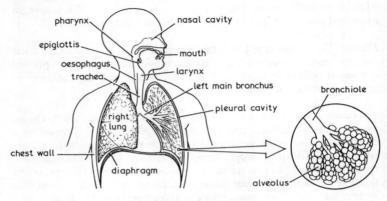

Fig. 1/6 Respiratory system

through the pulmonary veins to be passed on to the rest of the body, via the systemic circulation, where the oxygen is given up in the tissues. At the same time, deoxygenated haemoglobin and carbon dioxide are brought back to the lungs so that the carbon dioxide can be passed out from the capillaries through the air sac walls. (Note that except in the pulmonary circulation, arteries carry bright red 'oxygenated' blood to the tissues and veins carry dark red 'deoxygenated' blood from them.)

The expired air contains about 16 per cent oxygen (thus having lost about five per cent to the body) and now contains an increase of about four per cent of carbon dioxide.

The thoracic cavity which contains the lungs surrounded by a serous membrane, the *pleura*, is expanded by the action of muscles which raise the ribs and also by the depression of the *diaphragm*, a muscular sheet that separates the thorax from the abdomen. Expiration is usually achieved passively by an elastic 'recoil'. The respiratory cycle is mainly under the control of the respiratory centres of the brain which monitor the carbon dioxide levels in the circulating blood, but it is also under voluntary control for periods, e.g. breath-holding and during speech.

DIGESTIVE SYSTEM (Fig. 1/7)

This system is concerned with the taking in (ingestion) of food and its preparation and breakdown for assimilation by the body. The *alimentary canal* is comprised of the mouth, pharynx and oesophagus above the diaphragm and the stomach, the small intestine (duodenum, jejunum and ileum) and large intestine (colon) and rectum below it.

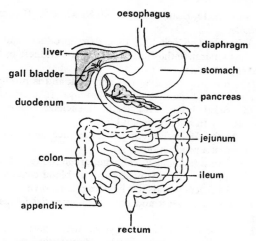

Fig. 1/7 Digestive system (below the diaphragm)

Food

The body requires food for growth and repair and also to provide fuel for heat and energy. Foods contain a variety of important components.

1. Proteins. These are found in meat, eggs, cheese, and beans, and can be broken down to their basic *amino acids* which are important body-tissue building and repair materials.

2. Carbohydrates (sugars, starches). These provide the body with heat and energy. Once assimilated they may be stored in the liver and muscles in the form of *glycogen*.

3. Fats. These are contained in milk, butter, animal fat, olive oil, and other fats, and, like carbohydrates, are fuel foods. Fat may be stored in the body in the adipose tissue.

4. Mineral salts. The body tissues require adequate amounts of certain basic elements, in the form of soluble salts, including sodium, potassium, calcium, magnesium, phosphorus, sulphur, iron and iodine plus minute amounts of manganese, copper, zinc, and other other trace elements.

5. Vitamins. These are essential food factors required for life, health and growth. Vitamins A, D, E and K are *fat-soluble* while B_1, B-complex and C are *water-soluble*.

Vitamin A is found in fish liver oils, dairy products and carrots. A deficiency of this vitamin in the diet leads to night-blindness and a 'dry-eye' condition (xerophthalmia).

Vitamin D is found in fish liver oils and milk and is produced by the exposure of the skin to sun or ultraviolet rays. It is essential for the formation of sound bones and teeth. Deficiency causes soft-bone deformities (rickets) in infants and children.

Vitamin E, found in green vegetables, lettuce and wheat-germ, is essential for normal reproduction.

Vitamin K is found in spinach, cabbage, green foods and some cereal, and is necessary for the formation of a blood-coagulation factor (prothrombin). Deficiency leads to a bleeding (haemorrhagic) tendency.

Vitamin B_1, found in yeast and cereals, is essential for carbohydrate metabolism.

Vitamin B-complex is found in liver, yeast, wheat-germ and egg-yolk; a deficiency may lead to skin inflammation (dermatitis), cracks round the lips and nose, eye infections and anaemia.

Vitamin C is found in fruit, especially citrus fruits, tomatoes, black-currants and fresh vegetables; it is essential for the formation of connective tissues and their products, e.g. teeth and bones. Deficiency causes *scurvy* with bleeding from the mucous membranes and gingivae, beneath the skin and in the joint cavities with progressive anaemia, weakness and death if not treated over a period of many weeks.

6. *Water.* This is essential for the processes of digestion and excretion, to maintain the fluid balances of the tissues and to assist in temperature regulation (e.g. sweating).

Digestion
Digestion is the process of mechanically and chemically breaking down food into simple compounds suitable for absorption into the body. The process may be divided into four stages:

1. *Ingestion and mastication.* Food is taken into the mouth and chewed (masticated) between the teeth, being held there by the action of the lips, tongue and cheeks. As the food is crushed and broken up it is mixed with saliva from the salivary glands which have been stimulated by the sight, smell and taste of the food. *Saliva*, a mixed secretion from the three pairs of salivary glands and the small mucous glands of the mucous membrane, contains the digestive enzyme, *ptyalin*, which converts starches to sugars. (An enzyme is an agent, usually a protein, that has the property of

30

accelerating a chemical reaction.) The saliva is mixed with the food, thoroughly moistening it and lubricating it for swallowing. The mass of food is now moulded into a ball or *bolus*.

2. *Deglutition* (swallowing). This has three stages, the first voluntary, the other two involuntary.

(a) The bolus is placed at the back of the tongue, the teeth are brought together and the tongue raised upwards and backwards to project the food into the pharynx.

(b) The bolus is now passed rapidly through the upper part of the pharynx, which is the region common to both the respiratory and digestive passages. The tongue remains in position to prevent the food returning to the mouth. The soft palate is raised to touch the back of the pharynx and stop the food from entering the nose. The larynx is raised up until it lies under the protection of the epiglottis at the base of the tongue and respiration is inhibited for a moment so that the food cannot enter the trachea. The bolus is gripped by the constrictor muscles of the pharynx and passed into the oesophagus (gullet).

(c) The oesophagus is a muscular tube that conducts the food down to the stomach by a wave of muscular contraction (*peristalsis*) that is partly aided by gravity. The food is thus carried through the chest and down through the diaphragm into the abdomen, entering the stomach through a ring of muscle, the *cardiac sphincter*, that acts as a valve guarding the entrance.

3. *Digestion and absorption*. In the stomach the food is mixed with the gastric juices by the muscular contractions of the stomach walls. *Gastric juice* is secreted by special cells in the stomach lining. It is highly acid and contains special enzymes including *pepsin*, *rennin* and *lipase* which act upon the proteins and fats.

At intervals the acid contents of the stomach, the *chyme*, are released into the upper part of the small intestine, the *duodenum*. The duodenal contents soon become alkaline by the action of digestive fluids brought to the duodenum by ducts from the liver and pancreas. *Bile* from the liver is alkaline and also emulsifies fats. *Pancreatic juice* contains the enzymes *amylase*, *lipase* and *trypsin* which act on carbohydrates, fats and proteins respectively. *Succus entericus*, the intestinal juice secreted by tiny glands in the small intestine wall also contains *erepsin*, an enzyme which acts upon proteins and *invertase, maltase* and *lactase* which deal with sugars. The fluid food is passed along the intestine by peristaltic waves of muscular contraction which are preceded by corresponding waves of relaxation. By now all the usable food material has been broken down to its final state ready for absorption. This takes place through the walls of the small intestine (duodenum, jejunum and ileum). The walls are raised into tiny

31

finger-like processes, *villi*, which greatly increase the absorbing surface of the intestine. The villi are well served with blood capillaries and lymphatics, here called *lacteals*. The food products are taken either directly into the blood stream and carried straight to the liver for storage or further chemical processes or, in the case of fat, into the lacteal and hence into the lymphatic system and on to the general circulation.

4. Excretion. The unusable residue and waste products pass on into the large intestine where water and salts are removed and the more solid *faeces* are passed into the *rectum* for elimination through the *anus*.

(The term *excretion* means the discharge of waste materials from the body. The kidneys filter the blood and eliminate water, salts and other end-products of metabolism via the urine. The lungs excrete carbon dioxide and water and can eliminate inhalation anaesthetic agents. The skin excretes water and salts in the perspiration. The saliva can also excrete certain materials, e.g. mercury and lead, in cases of poisoning.)

NERVOUS SYSTEM

This is the communication system of the body. The brain, spinal cord and nerves are composed of nerve cells and their processes. Each nerve cell or *neurone* has many processes, *dendrites*, for collecting impulses, and a single process, the *axon*, for passing the impulse on from the cell body. The nervous system is composed of millions of linked neurones.

The system is divided into two sub-systems: the *central nervous system* (the brain, spinal cord and peripheral nerves) and the *autonomic nervous system* (the sympathetic and parasympathetic systems).

Central nervous system
Brain. This is the control centre for the whole body. It weighs about two per cent of the total body-weight and requires a litre of oxygenated blood every minute. Lack of oxygen for more than ten seconds results in loss of consciousness and if this deficiency continues for more than four minutes permanent brain damage will result. The brain is covered by the vascular *meninges* and these in turn are covered by a tough protective membrane, the *dura mater*.

Peripheral nervous system. This system connects the brain to all parts of the body. It is composed of two kinds of nerves, the *efferent nerves* which carry messages from the brain and spinal cord to various parts of the body, e.g. motor impulses to voluntary muscles; and *afferent nerves* which relay messages back to the brain for interpretation, e.g. sensations of pain or temperature changes from the skin.

Cranial nerves. These originate from the brain within the cranium. Some are *sensory*, some are *motor* and some are *mixed* nerves.

	Name	Type	Distribution and Function
1st	Olfactory	Sensory	Olfactory mucous membrane of the nose – SMELL
2nd	Optic	Sensory	Retina of eye – SIGHT
3rd	Oculomotor	Motor	Eyeball muscles
4th	Trochlear	Motor	Eyeball muscles
5th	Trigeminal	Mixed	Sensory to forehead, face, nose, mouth, teeth, etc; three branches: (i) ophthalmic, (ii) maxillary, (iii) mandibular
			Motor to muscles of mastication
6th	Abducens	Motor	Eyeball muscle
7th	Facial	Mixed	Sensory to anterior two-thirds of tongue – TASTE
			Motor to muscles of facial expression
8th	Auditory	Sensory	From the cochlea – HEARING. From the semicircular canals via the vestibular nerve – BALANCE
9th	Glosso-pharyngeal	Mixed	Sensory from the tongue – TASTE
			Motor to muscles of the pharynx
10th	Vagus	Mixed	Supplies the pharynx, larynx, trachea, bronchi, lungs, heart, stomach oesophagus and upper part of the intestine
11th	Accessory	Motor	Muscles of pharynx, larynx and muscles in the neck and shoulder
12th	Hypoglossal	Motor	Muscles of the tongue

The fifth and seventh nerves (the trigeminal and facial) are described in more detail in Chapter 2, pages 54 and 56.

Spinal cord. This lies within the vertebral canal and gives off 31 pairs of mixed spinal nerves which serve all parts of the body, either by direct communication with the brain or by reflex action. Reflex actions are involuntary movements, e.g. when the hand is pricked with a pin it is withdrawn rapidly without conscious thought.

Autonomic nervous system
This system is connected with the brain and central nervous system but is devoted to involuntary action which takes place in, for example, the intestines, the blood vessels, heart and lungs. The sympathetic and parasympathetic systems which together make up the autonomic system, work in opposition to one another, the action of one stimulating an organ

33

while the action of the other inhibits it, e.g. the heart rate and force are increased by the sympathetic and decreased by the parasympathetic; the bronchi are relaxed by the sympathetic and contracted by the para-sympathetic. In this way a precise adjustment or tone between activity and rest can be maintained.

Sympathetic system. This is a double chain of ganglia (groups of nerve cells) which lie in front of the vertebral column from the base of the skull to the pelvis and send branches to the heart, blood vessels, stomach, intestines, muscles and skin and most other organs.

Parasympathetic system. This operates through the 3rd, 7th, 9th and 10th cranial nerves to the eyes, salivary glands, and all over the body via the vagus nerve and through the sacral region of the spinal cord. Its distribution is similar to the sympathetic.

Chapter Two

DENTAL ANATOMY AND PHYSIOLOGY

Study note: The study of the shape of individual teeth and the bones of the upper and lower jaw is greatly simplified by referring to the actual structures. We would advise the student to collect and sterilise a set of extracted human teeth for study; to examine either a plastic or dried skull; to examine her own dental structure in a mirror as well as those of patients undergoing treatment; and to feel the movement of her own jaws, i.e. the contraction of the facial and masticatory muscles and the temporo-mandibular joint.

TEETH

These are hard, mineralised structures which are set in bony sockets in the upper and lower jaws. Their main function is to masticate food and prepare it for swallowing. They also play an important part in the growth and final contour of the lower half of the face and are required for the clear articulation of certain sounds in speech.

A tooth consists of two main parts: the *crown* which is the part visible in the mouth and the *root* (or roots) which is the part set in the jaw. Where the crown and the root join, the tooth is usually constricted into the *neck* (the cervix or *cervical region*) (Fig. 2/1).

There are four main types of teeth: *incisors* or cutting teeth at the front of the mouth; *canines* ('eye teeth' or 'teeth such as dogs have'), at the corners of the mouth, which are used for gripping and tearing; *premolars* (bicuspids) which are not present in the child's primary dentition and *molars* or millstone teeth at the back of the mouth.

The teeth are set into the upper (maxillary) and lower (mandibular) alveolar processes (the special tooth-supporting bone) in curved arcades or *dental arches*.

Each tooth has four surrounding surfaces and a working edge or surface: *mesial*, nearest to the median plane; *distal*, furthest away from the median plane; *labial* or *buccal* nearest to the lips or cheek; *lingual* nearest to the

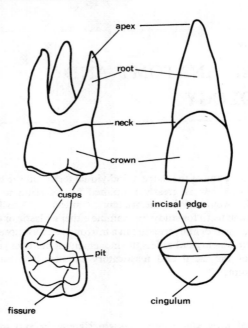

Fig. 2/1 External anatomy of teeth: (left) an upper molar; (right) an upper incisor

tongue (in the upper jaw the term *palatal*, nearest to the palate, is generally used instead of *lingual*); *occlusal*, the working surface of molars and premolars; *incisal edge*, the cutting edge of incisors (Figs. 2/2 and 2/3). The *proximal* surfaces are those which lie against the adjacent teeth in the same arch, i.e. the mesial and distal.

Cusps are the raised mounds on the occlusal surfaces of molars and premolars and raised lines are called *ridges*. *Fissures* are the line crevices between cusps. Small pin-point depressions are called *pits*. The *contact area* of a tooth is where it touches the surface of an adjacent tooth in the same arch. A *cingulum* is the raised ridge prominent only on the palatal surface of upper incisors.

Each tooth is made up of four tissues, enamel, dentine, dental pulp and cementum (Fig. 2/4) and is supported by the periodontal structures of the tooth socket.

Enamel. This is the hard, translucent, mineralised, insensitive material which covers the anatomical crown of the tooth. It is the hardest tissue in

Fig. 2/2 Tooth surfaces in the maxilla

Fig. 2/3 Tooth surfaces in the mandible

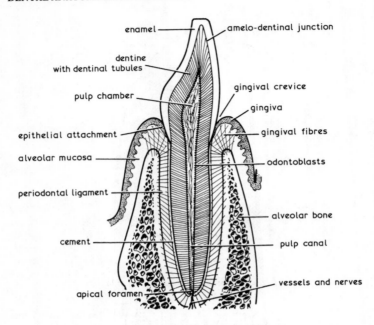

Fig. 2/4 A tooth and its component tissues

the body, composed mainly of calcium and phosphorus in the form of *hydroxyapatite* and containing only some one per cent of organic material. It is formed in microscopic *prisms* (or *rods*) joined by weaker *interprismatic substance* along which the enamel may be sheared or fractured mechanically during cavity preparation. It is thickest at the occlusal surface of the teeth.

Dentine. This is the yellowish, tough, slightly elastic material which forms the bulk of the tooth. In the crown it lies just beneath the enamel which it contacts at the *amelo-dentinal junction*. Dentine is mineralised but has about a 20 per cent organic content. It is traversed by fine *tubules* each containing a *fibril* or thread from the outer layer of pulpal cells, the *odontoblasts*. Thus dentine is sensitive, and with the pulp can react to moderate stimulation or injury but is vulnerable to strong chemicals or excessive heating during cavity preparation, etc. (Note: the *ivory* of an elephant's tusk is dentine.)

Dental pulp. This is the 'nerve' or soft tissue which occupies the pulp chamber of the crown and the root canal(s) within the dentine. The root canal communicates with the *peri-apical* (around the tip of the root) tissues through the *apical foramen* of the tooth. The pulp contains nerve fibres, blood vessels, lymphatics and connective tissue and is surrounded at its junction with the dentine by the continuous layer of odontoblasts. The pulp gives the tooth vitality, nutrition and sensitivity; in the embryonic stages it is formative and forms the dentine; and it plays a defensive role in repairing damaged dentine by calcification and the formation of *secondary dentine* within the pulp chamber. The pulp gets smaller with age.

Cementum. This is the thin layer of material which covers the anatomical root of the tooth. It resembles bone in composition and serves to attach the periodontal fibres to the tooth. It protects the underlying dentine, reacts to compensate for occlusal stresses and strains by changing in thickness and may transmit a little nutrition to the tooth from the periodontal tissues.

Periodontal membrane. This is the ligament which attaches the tooth to the walls of the socket formed around it by the alveolar bone. It is composed of strong connective tissue fibres together with numerous cells and blood vessels, lymphatics and nerves. At the neck of the tooth these tissues merge with those of the gingivae and the periosteum of the bone. The principal fibres of the periodontal membrane are described according to their function and the direction in which they run.

The free gingival fibres from the cervical cementum together with *vertical fibres* from the alveolar crest or socket margin pass into the gum next to the tooth to keep it in firm contact with the tooth. *Transeptal fibres* run from one tooth to its neighbour, interdentally, and help to maintain the arch. The *circular ligament* and *horizontal fibres* pass from the alveolar crest region to the cervical cementum and stabilise the tooth against lateral stress. (These important fibres are the first to disintegrate in the onset of periodontal disease.) Below this level the major part of the ligament is composed of *oblique fibres* that pass obliquely upwards from the cementum in the direction of the alveolar crest. All these fibres serve to stabilise and cushion the tooth against masticatory strains. The nerve endings are sensitive to pressure and pain and thus give a general awareness of which teeth are in contact during mastication and protect the dental apparatus from excessive pressure, e.g. on a stone.

The width of the various regions of the periodontal membrane varies according to occlusal stress and it becomes thinner with age as the cementum thickens.

ALVEOLAR BONE PROCESSES

These processes of the maxilla and mandible form the tooth sockets which are closely adapted to the shape of the roots. The socket walls are perforated by numerous foramina which transmit blood vessels and nerves to the periodontal membrane and the tooth. The lining of the socket wall to which the periodontal fibres are attached is composed of slightly denser bone, the *lamina dura*, which can be identified on an intra-oral radiograph. The alveolar bone adapts and remodels gradually in response to functional pressures.

THE GINGIVA

This is also called the 'gum' and is that part of the oral mucosa which surrounds the teeth. In health it is pale pink, slightly stippled on the surface and in close contact with the tooth. The *free gingiva* is separated from the tooth surface by the shallow *gingival crevice*. At the base of this crevice there is a firm *epithelial attachment* between the epithelial tissues and the tooth surface. (This attachment is destroyed in the first stages of pocket formation – see Chapter 11.) The interdental space is occupied by the *interdental papilla* of gingival tissue. The gingivae have a good blood supply and contain a high proportion of connective tissue.

ORAL MUCOSA

This lines the whole oral cavity and is composed basically of two layers: the *epithelium* and the underlying *connective tissues*. It contains numerous tiny mucous glands and is thickened in places of intensive masticatory wear, e.g. the palate (where it is raised in ridges, the *rugae*), and the gingivae. Over the surface of the tongue the mucosa is specialised to serve the sense of taste. The junction between the red margins of the lips and the external skin is called the *transitional zone*.

DEVELOPMENT OF THE TEETH AND JAWS

At an early stage in the development of the human embryo, the cells are differentiated into three layers: the *ectoderm*, which will form the external surface of the body and its derivatives including parts of the mouth, the salivary glands and enamel of the teeth and most of the central nervous system; the *endoderm* which gives rise to the alimentary canal and such things as the lungs and air passages; and the *mesoderm* which forms the remaining organs and tissues including the dentine, cementum and pulp of the teeth, the muscles and cardiovascular system.

The face and neck of the embryo begins to differentiate as early as five weeks in utero into the form of six primitive *visceral arches*, like those of a fish, in the wall of the foregut. The first of these arches, the *mandibular*, will go on to form the lower jaw, chin, the anterior two-thirds of the tongue and the muscles of mastication, carrying with it the mandibular division of the 5th trigeminal nerve. In addition, the maxilla, excluding the pre-maxilla, is developed from the maxillary processes of the mandibular arch. The second arch, the *hyoid*, forms the muscles of facial expression, etc, carrying with it the 7th facial nerve. The third arch forms the posterior part of the tongue and carries the 9th glossopharyngeal nerve fibres with it.

The tooth germ (Fig. 2/5) This begins to form by a proliferation of ectodermal cells in the primitive mouth at about six weeks in utero. The cells form a band, the *dental lamina*, around the jaw and at nine weeks little buds of cells appear, one for each primary tooth. These buds form into the bell-shaped *enamel organs* (which have an internal wall of enamel-forming cells, the *ameloblasts*) and stimulate the associated mesodermal cells to form *dental papillae* which will in turn form the dentine and dental pulp. Each tooth germ is contained inside a sac called the *dental follicle*. Offshoots from these tooth germs and a distal extension of the dental lamina make provision for the permanent tooth buds. Mineralisation of the teeth begins at about 18 weeks, so that at birth a considerable part of the deciduous teeth is already calcified.

Eruption of teeth. This is not fully understood. It may be due to blood pressure, root growth, changes in the bone of the alveolar process or even

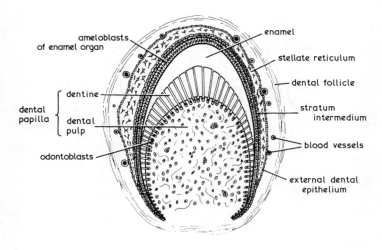

Fig. 2/5 A developing tooth

the influence of the 'ingrown' epithelial tissues trying to return to the surface. The tooth gradually rises to the surface and the epithelial remnants of the enamel organ (Nasmyth's membrane, the 'skin of the tooth') become attached to the surface epithelium at the gingival crevice as the tooth erupts into the mouth. This attachment recedes gradually until it rests on the amelo-cemental junction. Teeth commonly erupt before the apex of the root is fully formed and this is completed in conjunction with the formation of the final socket.

THE DENTITIONS (Figs. 2/6, 2/7 and 2/8)

There are two dentitions: the primary, deciduous or 'milk teeth' of the child (Fig. 2/6) and the permanent or secondary teeth (Fig. 2/7).

Primary dentition (Fig. 2/6)

This consists of 20 teeth, five in each quadrant: two incisors, one canine and two molars. They are small teeth, set vertically in the alveolus, with whiter enamel than the permanent teeth. They have relatively barrel-shaped crowns with large pulps and slender tapering roots. The permanent premolar tooth germs lie between the divergent roots of the molars. The upper 1st molar has three cusps while the upper 2nd molar has four cusps. The lower 1st molar has four cusps and the lower 2nd molar has five cusps.

Fig. 2/6 The primary teeth (primary dentition)

Eruption and Calcification Table for Primary Teeth

	Calcification				
	Begins (intra-uterine)	*Completed (after birth)*	*Tooth erupts*	*Resorption begins*	*Tooth shed*
1st incisor ⎫ 2nd incisor ⎭	18th week	18 months	{ 6 months { 8 months	3 years	7th year 8th year
1st molar	20th week	20 months	12 months	before	9th year
canine ⎫ 2nd molar ⎭	24th week	24 months	{ 18 months { 24 months	being shed	11th year 10th year

Permanent dentition (Fig. 2/7)

This consists of 32 teeth, eight in each quadrant: two incisors, one canine, two premolars and three molars.

Incisors. These are the chisel-shaped cutting teeth at the front of the mouth. They have one root and the crown is convex on the labial surface and concave on the palatal/lingual surface. The upper central incisor is larger than the others and may have a ridge on the palatal surface, near the cervical region, called the *cingulum.*

Canine tooth. This is also called the cuspid and is a strong, conical tooth more massive than an incisor, with a single root that is usually larger than any of the others in the mouth. The lower canine is smaller than the upper.

Fig. 2/7 The permanent teeth (permanent dentition)

43

Premolars. These are also called bicuspids and occupy a position between the canines and the molars. They have occlusal surfaces with cusps. The 1st upper premolar may have two roots but all the others have only one root. The lingual cusp on the lower 1st premolar is very small and care must be taken not to confuse this tooth with the canine.

Molars. These teeth have the largest occlusal surfaces; the upper molars have four cusps, the lower 1st molar has five cusps, the lower 2nd molar has four cusps and the lower 3rd molar has five cusps. The upper molar teeth each have three roots (mesio-buccal, disto-buccal and palatal) while the lower molars each have two roots (mesial and distal). The third molars, the 'wisdom teeth', may occasionally vary from this pattern of cusp and root numbers. Sometimes there is an additional palatal cusp on the upper first molars – the cusp of Carabelli.

Figure 2/8 illustrates how the primary and permanent dentitions overlap in the jaws.

Fig. 2/8 Orthopantomogram showing the mixed dentition in a child

Eruption and Calcification Table for Permanent Teeth
(after Aitchison)

		Tooth erupts (years)	Calcification	
			begins	completed
1.	1st incisor	7	for all teeth	
2.	2nd incisor	8	6 years before eruption	3 years after eruption
3.	canine	11	except for canine	
4.	1st premolar	9	and 3rd molar	
5.	2nd premolar	10	when calcification	
6.	1st molar	6	begins 9 years	canine and 3rd
7.	2nd molar	12	before	molar completely
8.	3rd molar	18–24	eruption	calcified upon eruption

THE JAWS

Maxillae (Figs. 2/9, 2/10 and 2/11)

These together form the left and right halves of the upper jaw. Each bone supports the upper teeth, forms the hard palate (in conjunction with the palatine bone) and helps to make up the floor of the orbit and the floor and lateral wall of the nasal cavity. The maxilla has a pyramid-shaped body with

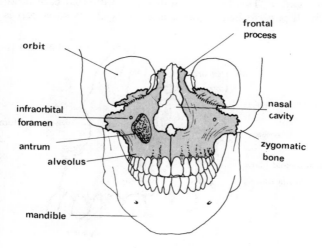

Fig. 2/9 Frontal aspect of the maxilla

45

four surfaces: anterior, posterior, nasal and orbital, and four processes: frontal, zygomatic, palatine and alveolar. The body of the maxilla encloses a large air cavity: the *maxillary air sinus* or *antrum*.

Maxillary sinus. This communicates with the nasal cavity and is lined with ciliated, respiratory epithelium. The floor of the sinus lies in close relationship to the roots of the 1st and 2nd upper molar teeth and in some cases a large sinus may relate to all the molars and premolars. (This fact must be borne in mind during infections or extraction of these teeth.) The posterior wall is perforated by the dental canals carrying posterior superior dental vessels and nerves to the molar teeth.

Orbital surface. This forms part of the floor of the orbit and has a groove running forwards which carries the infra-orbital nerve and artery down via the *infra-orbital canal* to the *infra-orbital foramen* to the surface of the face below the orbit (Fig. 2/10).

Anterior surface. This supports the cheek and carries three processes: the *frontal* which passes upwards on the medical aspect of the orbit and articulates with the frontal bone and the nasal bone; the *zygomatic* which articulates with the *zygomatic bone* (the cheek bone) and the *alveolar process* which supports the teeth.

Posterior surface. This bulges outwards and is directed backwards and laterally. It is perforated by the dental canals. At its lower part is the

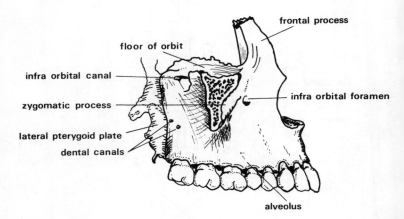

Fig. 2/10 Lateral aspect of the right maxilla

maxillary tuberosity, a rounded knob of bone that lies distally to the upper 3rd molar in the arch.

Nasal surface. This carries the opening of the antrum and forms part of the wall of the nasal cavity.

Palatal process (Fig. 2/11). This articulates in the mid-line with the opposite maxilla and with the palatal bone posteriorly to form the hard palate. The palate is grooved at its posterior part to provide a channel for the *greater palatine vessels and nerve* as they run forward from the *greater palatine foramen*. Immediately behind the incisor teeth lies the *incisive fossa* which transmits the *long sphenopalatine nerve* and the *sphenopalatine artery*.

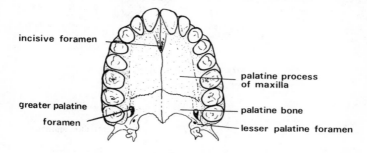

incisive foramen

palatine process of maxilla

greater palatine foramen

palatine bone

lesser palatine foramen

Fig. 2/11 Palatal aspect of the maxilla

Mandible (Figs. 2/12 and 2/13)
This is also called the lower jaw and is the largest and strongest bone of the face. It articulates on each side with the *glenoid fossa* of the temporal bone. It is formed of two parts: the horseshoe-shaped, curved, horizontal *body* and the two broad, flattened *rami* which project upwards from the posterior ends of the body.

Body. This is composed of right and left halves which are fused in the mid-line at the *symphysis menti*.

External surface of the body. At the mid-line the chin is formed by the triangular *mental protuberance*. The depression above this protuberance is the *incisive fossa*. The *external oblique* line runs upwards and backwards from the margin of the mental protuberance to become the anterior border of the ascending ramus. Below and between the premolar teeth the *mental foramen* transmits the mental nerve and vessels.

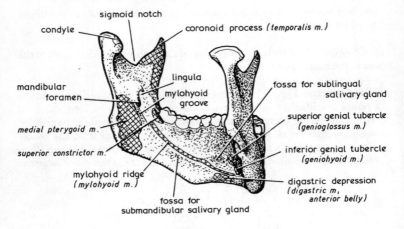

Fig. 2/12 The mandible from behind

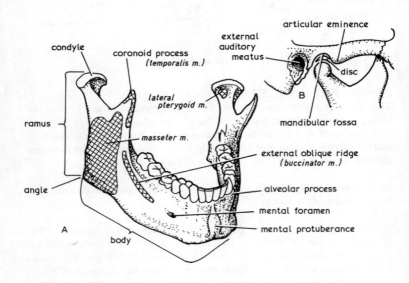

Fig. 2/13 The mandible from the front

Internal surface of the body. This is divided into two areas by the *mylohyoid ridge* which gives attachment to the mylohyoid muscle and runs obliquely down from behind the third molar to a point low down at the mid-line behind the symphysis menti. Just above this mid-line point are two pairs of small tubercles, the *genial tubercles*, which are the origin of the *genioglossus* and *geniohyoid* muscles. Below the mylohyoid line near the symphysis lies the hollow of the *digastric depression* which gives rise to the *anterior belly of the digastric muscle*. Below the posterior part of the mylohyoid ridge is the *submandibular fossa* for the submandibular salivary gland and above the anterior part of the ridge lies the *sublingual fossa* for the sublingual salivary gland.

Upper border of the body. This forms the alveolar process which supports the teeth. The *lower border* is thick, smooth and rounded and is continuous behind with the thin lower border of the ramus.

The ramus. This is a flattened quadrilateral shape with two surfaces, four borders and two processes.

External surface of the ramus. This is roughened by the insertion of the *masseter muscle*.

Internal surface of the ramus. In the centre of this surface, at the level of the occlusal plane of the molar teeth, is the *mandibular foramen* through which pass the inferior dental nerve and vessels into the mandibular canal. Guarding the front of the foramen is a tongue of bone, the *lingula*, which gives attachment for the *sphenomandibular ligament*. A shallow *mylohyoid groove* (for the mylohyoid nerve and vessels) runs downwards and forwards for a short distance. Below this groove is an area roughened by the attachment of the *medial pterygoid muscle*.

Borders of the ramus. The *inferior border* is thin and rounded and in continuity with the body in front. Its junction with the *posterior border* forms the angle of the mandible. This posterior border is rounded and smooth and is surrounded by the *parotid gland*. The *anterior border* is continuous with the external oblique line of the body. The *superior border* has two important processes separated by a notch, the *sigmoid notch*. The anterior process is the thin triangular *coronoid process* which carries the insertion of the *temporalis muscle* on its internal and anterior surfaces. The posterior process carries the *condyle* which has a broad, strong, rounded head on a thin neck and forms the joint surface which articulates with the temporal bone.

49

Temporomandibular joint (Fig. 2/13B)

This is a sliding-hinge joint which allows grinding movements of the jaws to take place. The *glenoid fossa* of the temporal bone is an oblong concavity bounded anteriorly by a raised *articular eminence*. As the body of the mandible moves downwards, the condyle slides forwards and downwards on to the eminence. The joint has a fibro-cartilaginous *disc* which is more firmly attached to the condyle than the fossa. The joint is protected by the *capsular ligament* around the joint, strengthened by internal and external *lateral ligaments* and further reinforced by the *sphenomandibular ligament* (spine of the sphenoid to the lingula) and *stylomandibular ligaments* (styloid process to the posterior border of the ramus above the angle of the jaw).

MUSCLES OF MASTICATION (Figs. 2/14 and 2/15)

Temporalis. This is a fan-shaped muscle. Its origin is the temporal fossa at the side of the cranium and its insertion the coronoid process of the mandible. It serves to elevate the mandible and also draw it backwards.

Masseter. This is a quadrilateral muscle in superficial and deep portions. It arises from the zygomatic arch and is inserted in the outer surface of the ramus of the mandible. It also serves to elevate the mandible.

(The action of these muscles and the movement of the temporo-mandibular joint can be felt by placing the fingers in the appropriate

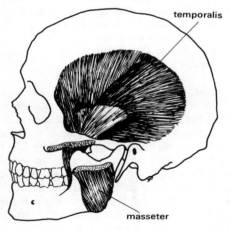

Fig. 2/14 Superficial muscles of mastication

positions at the side of the head while opening and closing the mouth and clenching the teeth.)

Medial pterygoid. This is a thick quadrilateral muscle with its origin in the medial surface of the pterygoid plate of the sphenoid and its insertion in the lower part of the internal surface of the ramus of the mandible. Its action is to elevate the mandible and also to protrude the chin.

Lateral pterygoid. This is a short cone-shaped muscle originating from the infra-temporal surface of the greater wing of the sphenoid and the lateral surface of the pterygoid plate. Its insertion is the front of the neck of the condyle and the joint capsule and disc of the temporomandibular joint. Its purpose is to draw the condyle forwards and inwards for side-to-side chewing, to protrude the chin and also to assist in depressing the mandible (opening the jaws).

All four of these muscles of mastication are developed from the 1st branchial arch and receive their motor nerve supply from the mandibular division of the 5th trigeminal nerve.

Hyoid muscles. Apart from the lateral pterygoid, the muscles which depress the mandible are weak by comparison with the elevator muscles and are assisted by the force of gravity. They are associated with the *hyoid bone* which lies in the front of the neck below the mandible. The hyoid is acted

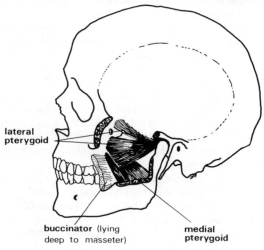

lateral
pterygoid

buccinator (lying
deep to masseter)

medial
pterygoid

Fig. 2/15 Deep muscles of mastication

51

upon by the *infrahyoid muscles* (to the sternum, etc) and by the *suprahyoid muscles* – the *digastric, mylohyoid* (the muscular floor of the mouth), *geniohyoid* and *stylohyoid*, the first three of which have attachments to the internal surface of the body of the mandible. Their action in depressing the mandible may be further assisted by the superficial skin muscle of the neck, the *platysma*.

In summary the possible movements of the mandible are: *protruding*; *elevating* to occlude the teeth; *retruding*; *depressing* to open the mouth, and *side to side* for chewing.

Mastication is also assisted by the actions of the *buccinator* muscle in the cheek and by the tongue.

The *buccinator* muscle of the wall of the cheek runs from the orbicularis oris in front to join the upper muscles of the pharynx at the *pterygo-mandibular raphe* which runs down from the region of the pterygoid plate to the mandible behind the third molar. Above and below, it arises from the outer surfaces of the alveolus opposite the molar teeth. It serves to press the cheek against the teeth and prevent food from collecting in the buccal *vestibule* (the oral space buccally and labially to the teeth) during mastication. This muscle is also used in blowing (*buccina* is Latin for a trumpet). Its motor nerve is the 7th or facial nerve.

Soft palate
The fold of tissue attached to the posterior border of the hard palate, which extends downwards and backwards and separates the nasal and oral parts of the pharynx. It can be moved by muscles to seal off the nasal cavity, e.g. during swallowing. The oral surface is covered with mucous membrane, and taste buds are present. The *uvula* is a small conical process extending from the mid-line of the free margin of the soft palate.

Tongue
This is a muscular organ associated with taste, swallowing and speech, and lies partly in the mouth and partly in the pharynx. The muscles of the root of the tongue are based on the hyoid bone and the genial tubercles of the mandible and other external muscles also join it from the styloid process, the palate and the pharynx. The motor nerve of the tongue muscles is the 12th or hypoglossal nerve.

The mucosa of the upper surface, sides and tip of the anterior two-thirds of the tongue is in the form of specialised *papillae*: *filiform* papillae, small, fine and thread-like, *fungiform* papillae, larger, round and deep red and the *circumvallate* papillae which are 8 to 10 cup-shaped depressions in a V-shaped arrangement at the junction of the oral and pharyngeal parts of the tongue.

Taste buds are specialised nerve endings embedded in the papillae. The receptors sensitive to saltiness and sweetness lie mainly at the tip and front of the tongue, to sourness along the edges and to bitterness at the back of the tongue. The taste nerves for the anterior two-thirds are from the 7th facial nerve and the posterior third from the 9th glossopharyngeal nerve. (A further component of 'taste' is added by the smell of food carried to the olfactory nerve in the nose.)

Muscles of facial expression

The facial muscles surround the openings of the eyes, nose, mouth and ears and serve as constrictors or dilators. They are all developed from the 2nd branchial arch and are served by its nerve, the 7th facial nerve. Their finely balanced action serves to change the facial contours and express the emotions as in scowling, smiling, winking and so on.

The mouth is surrounded by a broad, flat ring of muscle, the *orbicularis oris* and bands of muscle converge to join the angle of the mouth like the spokes of a wheel. The *zygomaticus* serves to raise, the *risorius* to draw back and the *depressor angularis* to lower the corner of the mouth in smiling or grinning or to turn the corners of the mouth down. Further groups of muscles attached to the mid-line of the lips (e.g. *levator labii superioris* in the upper, *mentalis* in the lower) serve to move these sections independently and to purse and pout the lips.

SALIVARY GLANDS

Parotid gland. This, the largest salivary gland, is wrapped around the posterior border of the ramus of the mandible and its associated structures. (It is the gland that commonly swells up in mumps.) It produces thin, serous saliva which is transmitted to the mouth through the parotid duct, *Stenson's duct*, which penetrates the buccinator muscle and opens opposite the second upper molar tooth.

Submandibular gland. This lies in the submandibular fossa on the inner surface of the body of the mandible and rests partially on the mylohyoid muscle. It produces a muco-serous saliva which is conducted forward through the submandibular duct (*Wharton's duct*) which opens at the *sublingual papilla* at one side of the *lingual fraenum* (the mid-line fold of mucosa beneath the tongue).

Sublingual gland. This is the smallest of the three main salivary glands and lies just beneath the mucosa of the floor of the mouth in the sublingual fossa of the body of the mandible. It produces a mainly thick, mucous saliva which passes straight into the mouth through some 10 to 20 sublingual ducts which open near the submandibular duct under the tongue.

The secretory, *secretomotor*, nerves for the salivary glands arise in the *salivatory centre* of the brain. They pass to the parotid gland via the 9th glossopharyngeal nerve, the tympanic branch fibres joining the *auriculotemporal nerve* which serves the area. The secretomotor nerves to the submandibular and sublingual glands are carried by a branch of the 7th facial nerve, the *chorda tympani*, via the *lingual nerve*.

Mucous glands. Those of the oral mucosa are numerous and all produce their addition to the saliva in the oral cavity.

In summary, the functions of saliva are: in *digestion* (it contains ptyalin); the *lubrication* of the food bolus; its *cleansing* action (removing food particles from the teeth); its *antibacterial* action used for protection, and its *buffer action* which stabilises changes in the acid/alkali balance of the mouth.

NERVE SUPPLY OF THE TEETH AND ORAL TISSUES

The nerves supplying this region are the 5th trigeminal, the 7th facial, 9th glossopharyngeal and the 12th hypoglossal cranial nerves.

Note: Please refer to page 153 for the Table of nerve supply to the individual teeth and surrounding structures (together with local anaesthesia used).

Trigeminal nerve (5th)
This is the largest cranial nerve. It is sensory for the face, scalp, mouth, teeth and nose, and motor to the muscles of mastication. It has a large sensory root and a smaller motor root and is divided into three main branches or divisions: the *ophthalmic*, the *maxillary* and the *mandibular*.

Ophthalmic nerve. This enters the orbit through the superior orbital fissure and divides into three branches, the *lacrimal*, *frontal* and *nasociliary* nerves. It is sensory to the eye, to the skin of the nose, forehead, eyelids and scalp and also part of the nasal mucosa. The frontal nerve passes through the *supra-orbital notch*.

Maxillary nerve. This leaves the cranium through the *foramen rotundum*, crosses the *pterygopalatine fossa* and enters the orbit via the *inferior orbital fissure*. It then passes into the infra-orbital groove and is transmitted through the infra-orbital foramen to the surface of the cheek.

In the pterygopalatine fossa it gives off three branches:

The zygomatic nerve. This enters the zygomatic bone and sends branches to the temporal fossa and to the skin of the cheek via the zygomatic-facial foramen.

The ganglionic nerve. This supplies the *sphenopalatine ganglion*, which is linked with the facial nerve and sends branches mainly to the palate, nose and pharynx. The *greater palatine nerve* descends through the greater palatine foramen and runs forward to serve the mucosa of the hard palate and adjacent gingivae. The *long sphenopalatine nerve* descends through the incisive fossa to serve the palatal mucosa behind the incisor teeth.

The posterior superior dental nerve. Branches from this nerve pass into the posterior surface of the maxilla to run in the canals in the wall of the sinus on their way to join the *middle superior dental* branches. Together they serve the lining of the sinus, the nearby molar and premolar teeth and their associated periodontal structures and cheek mucosa.

In the infra-orbital canal the maxillary nerve gives off the *middle superior dental* and *anterior superior dental* branches. The former serves the upper teeth in communication with the posterior superior dental nerve branches. The anterior branch passes through a sinuous canal in the anterior wall of the sinus and its branches serve the incisor and canine teeth and the floor of the nasal cavity.

The maxillary nerve finally passes through the infra-orbital foramen and gives off its terminal branches: *palpebral* to the lower eyelid, *nasal* to the nose and *labial* to the cheek, upper lip and local oral mucosa.

Mandibular nerve. The sensory root of this nerve is joined by the small motor root as it leaves the *foramen ovale* deep to the lateral pterygoid muscle.

The anterior trunk. This gives off motor branches to the muscles of mastication, the *medial pterygoid*, *lateral pterygoid*, *temporal* and *masseteric* nerves. It also gives off a sensory branch, the *buccal* nerve, which supplies the mucosa lining the cheek and the posterior buccal surface of the mandibular alveolar mucosa.

The posterior trunk. This divides into three branches: the *auriculotemporal* nerve which runs backwards behind the mandibular joint, communicates with the 7th facial nerve and serves the region of the ear, the joint, the parotid gland and the temporal skin, the *lingual* nerve which passes forwards to serve the mucous membrane of the anterior two-thirds of the tongue, the floor of the mouth and the lingual surface of the mandibular gingivae, and the *inferior dental* nerve. This gives off a small *mylohyoid* branch to the mylohyoid muscle and the anterior belly of the digastric muscle before it enters the mandibular foramen to run in the mandibular canal of the body of the mandible, giving off further branches to the molar and premolar teeth and their periodontal structures and associated buccal mucosa. At the mental foramen the *mental* nerve emerges to serve the skin and mucosa of the lip while the *incisive* nerve runs on in the bone to serve the incisor and canine teeth and their associated structures.

Facial nerve (7th)
This is the nerve of the second or hyoid arch and serves the muscles forming it including the muscles of the face, ear and scalp. Its terminal branches fan out from the borders of the parotid gland: the *postauricular*, the *temporal*, the *zygomatic*, the *buccal*, the *mandibular* and the *cervical*. The *chorda tympani* transmits secretomotor fibres on their way to the submandibular and sublingual glands and also carries taste sensory fibres from the anterior two-thirds of the tongue.

Glossopharyngeal nerve (9th)
This has sensory branches from the pharynx, tonsils and the posterior third of the tongue. It is secretomotor to the parotid gland and motor to the *stylopharyngeus*, a muscle of the pharynx.

Hypoglossal nerve (12th)
This is the motor nerve of the tongue serving styloglossus, hyoglossus, geniohyoid, genioglossus muscles and the intrinsic muscle fibres of that organ.

BLOOD SUPPLY TO THE TEETH AND ORAL TISSUES (Fig. 2/16)

The main arteries of the head and neck are the two *common carotid* arteries which divide into the *internal* and *external carotids* at the level of the thyroid cartilage of the larynx, the former going on to supply the inner parts of the cranium and orbit.

External carotid artery
This passes upwards through the neck giving off branches until it terminates at its final divisions within the structure of the parotid gland, level with the neck of the condyle. There are eight branches: the *superior thyroid*, *lingual*, *facial*, *occipital*, *ascending pharyngeal*, *posterior auricular*, *superficial temporal* and *maxillary* arteries.

The blood supply of the teeth is mainly from the lingual and maxillary arteries and most of their branches run on similar courses to the nerves, as also do the veins.

Lingual artery. This runs forward in a loop on the constrictor muscle of the pharynx in close association with the hypoglossal nerve at times and then rises to run on the inferior surface of the tongue near the mid-line, now accompanied by the lingual nerve. It serves the tongue and the floor of the mouth.

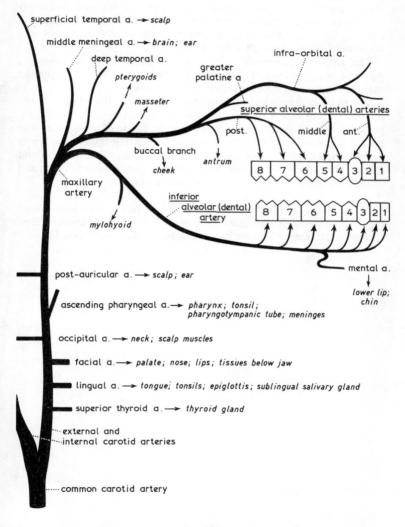

Fig. 2/16 Blood supply to the jaws, teeth and adjacent tissues

Maxillary artery. This arises deep to the neck of the condyle of the mandible and passes in relationship to the lateral pterygoid muscle on its way to the pterygomandibular fossa. Its first or mandibular part gives off branches to the ear and the brain (*meningeal* artery), before the *inferior dental* artery descends to the mandibular foramen, giving off the *mylohyoid* branch, and entering the mandibular canal to accompany the inferior dental nerve to serve the teeth and mental foramen region.

The second or pterygoid part of the maxillary artery has *temporal*, *pterygoid*, *masseteric* and *buccal* branches which closely follow the similar branches of the mandibular nerve to their muscles.

The third or pterygopalatine part has several more branches of dental importance. Branches of the *posterior superior dental* artery enter the posterior surface of the maxilla and serve the lining of the antrum, the premolar and molar teeth and the alveolar process. The *infra-orbital* artery has branches to the incisor and canine region. The *greater palatine* and *sphenopalatine* arteries descend through the greater palatine foramen and incisive fossa of the maxilla to serve the palatal mucosa.

Facial artery. This supplies tissues which include the muscles of facial expression, the sublingual gland, the soft palate and tonsil area and is of special dental interest because it supplies the labial arteries to the lips.

Chapter Three

BACTERIOLOGY AND PATHOLOGY

Bacteriology is the science which deals with micro-organisms and pathology is the study of diseases and their effects on the functions of the body.

BACTERIOLOGY

Bacteria (Fig. 3/1)

These are microscopic, single-celled organisms that are classified at the lower limit of the scale of living things. In favourable conditions they multiply by simple cell division. There are many different species of bacteria and they can be identified in the laboratory because of their different sizes and shapes, by the way they grow in colonies on special nutrient materials (culture media) and in the way they can be stained with special dye solutions.

Viruses

A virus is an extremely minute body often several hundred times smaller than a bacterium and thus invisible under the most powerful optical microscope and able to pass easily through the finest bacteria-stopping filters. They multiply inside the cells of the infected host. Rabies, smallpox and the common cold are all examples of diseases caused by viruses.

Saprophytes and parasites

Bacteria are found to be widely distributed in nature for they exist in vast numbers in soil, water, air and in all decaying organic matter. Those called collectively *saprophytes* exist on dead material, while *parasites* grow on living tissues. Some bacteria can adapt to exist in both situations. Like plants they will grow faster in ideal conditions. Each organism may then divide every 20 minutes and thus one cell could produce many millions in the course of a single day. Variations of temperature, oxygen level, available food and moisture will all affect this phenomenal growth rate.

Fig. 3/1 Bacterial types

When very unfavourable conditions arise some bacteria, e.g. the tetanus bacillus (the organism that causes tetanus or 'lockjaw'), can form *spores* which are tiny seed-like granules surrounded by a dense protective capsule. These spores can survive in boiling water (100°C) for almost an hour and still be capable of commencing new growth when they reach favourable conditions once more.

Pathogens

Only a small group of bacteria are able to cause disease in man and these are called *pathogens*. Pathogenic organisms produce powerful poisons called *toxins* which can give rise to the symptoms of the disease. *Endotoxins* tend to affect the tissues near to the infecting source and may be produced by the body of the organism itself after it has died. *Exotoxins*, on the other hand, can affect parts of the body that are some distance away from the site of the originating bacteria, e.g. in diphtheria the infecting organisms remain in the nasopharynx, but the exotoxins, getting into the circulation, can cause heart failure or nervous paralysis of the limbs. Common *pyogenic* (pus-forming) wound infections are caused by such organisms as staphylococcus and streptococcus.

Staphylococci. These are spherical bodies of about 1 micron (0.001mm) in diameter which divide in every plane and are thus arranged typically in grape-like clusters. Three types are known: *Staphylococcus aureus*, *Staphylococcus albus* and *Staphylococcus citreus*, so named because they produce golden, white and lemon-yellow colonies respectively when grown in the laboratory. *Staphylococcus aureus* is the most virulent and is responsible for boils, skin abscesses and other superficial infections. If it manages to spread to deeper tissues or enter the bloodstream it can cause such things as bone marrow infection (osteomyelitis) or generalised blood infection (septicaemia).

Streptococci. These are also spherical bodies of a similar size, but as they divide repeatedly in the same plane they are arranged characteristically in chains, like beads on a string. They can be subclassified as haemolytic, non-haemolytic or viridans because of their varying ability to dissolve red blood cells in a special laboratory culture medium. *Streptococcus haemolyticus* is present in the nose and throat of many people and is a potential source of infection to themselves as well as the other people with whom they come in contact. This is one of the reasons why surgeons wear masks when operating. This organism can infect wounds and cause abscesses or it may give rise to more spreading and generalised infections as in scarlet fever, pneumonia or middle ear infections. Of particular interest is *Streptococcus viridans* for it may be found in dental abscesses and is thought to have a link with certain kinds of infection of the inner surface of the heart and its valves (bacterial endocarditis). Non-haemolytic streptococci give rise to infections similar but less severe than those caused by the other classes.

PATHOLOGY

Protective mechanisms of the body

Countless numbers of bacteria live normally on the human body surfaces: on the skin, in the hair, in the mouth, nose and throat. They are constantly present in the air that is breathed in and in all food that is eaten. Several species of organisms are in permanent residence in the intestines and some even manufacture valuable nutritive materials for the body. Most of these organisms would cause infection and disease if they were able to penetrate the body's defensive system.

The human body has several protective barriers and mechanisms to resist invasion by pathogenic organisms. An intact skin and to a lesser extent an intact mucous membrane will shield the body against most bacteria. In addition sweat and other skin secretions all tend to wash away and discourage the growth of organisms. Tears, nasal secretions and saliva also have this constant cleaning action and many of these surface secretions contain a substance, lysozyme, which has a strong bactericidal effect. The gastric juices are strongly acid and capable of destroying most bacteria ingested in food. The lungs and respiratory tract are coated with a layer of sticky mucus which is constantly being moved, by specialised epithelial cells, against the incoming breath and thus carries any potential irritant or infection back to the throat where it is swallowed and dealt with by the gastric juices.

Immunity. This is a term used to describe an individual's general bodily resistance to infection. This may be *natural immunity* where a species, race or individual is resistant to a particular pathogen (e.g. man does not catch distemper from a dog) or it may be an *acquired immunity* as when recovery from a single attack of a disease gives life-long protection from a second attack (e.g. diphtheria, measles) by the production of *antibodies* in the blood.

Infection

Infection occurs when there is a successful invasion of the body by living pathogenic organisms with consequent damage to the host. The infecting organism can be transmitted to a human being in several ways:

1. By direct or indirect contact
2. By droplets or airborne infection
3. By being swallowed
4. By an insect or animal contact.

An organism's capacity to overcome the body's defences and invade the host depends upon its virulence, the power of the toxins it can produce, the numbers of bacteria that are present at the point of infection and the exact portal of entry. The host defences will be able to protect a small, shallow scratch more easily than a deep, jagged wound or an extensive burn.

Acute inflammation

This is the rapid reaction of the tissues to an irritant (bacterial, chemical, physical) which causes an injury that is not severe enough to kill them. Chemicals from the damaged cells go into the circulation and cause an urgent local, and later a general alarm reaction. The small blood vessels and capillaries adjacent to the wound become dilated and make the surrounding skin and tissues red and hot, then fluid and cells exude from these dilated vessels and swelling occurs. The sensory nerves to the area are stimulated by the toxins and the increasing pressure of the inflammatory exudate and give the sensation of throbbing pain. The structures and organs in the region all suffer an impairment of function.

Thus the cardinal signs and symptoms of acute inflammation are:
1. Heat
2. Redness
3. Swelling
4. Pain
5. Loss of function.

By this process fluids, specialised blood cells and complex chemical agents are brought to the area to localise and counteract the effects of the injury and attempt to resist infection and kill any invading organisms. The most important role in this cellular defence is played by the white cells (leucocytes) of blood, particularly the polymorphonuclear leucocyte which can move independently through the body tissues and actually engulf or 'eat' a dozen or more invading organisms and thus imprison and kill them. Masses of these white cells are attracted to an inflamed region. The products of this battle between the cells and organisms are gradually washed into the drainage system of the lymphatics and passed on to the nearest *lymphatic glands*. These glands may soon swell as a result of their increased activity.

The general bodily effects of the onset of acute inflammation are usually a feeling of chill and an attack of shivering, followed by a rise in temperature to 37.2°C or above, with an associated rise in the pulse rate and a general sensation of illness. Thus the body physically aids the defensive mechanisms by increasing the speed of the general circulation and the passage of blood to the damaged part, by making the inflamed region painful and difficult to use so that it is rested and helped to recover, and by making the host feel unwell and less inclined to squander his general strength. At the same time the rise in body temperature helps to increase general cellular activity. (Normal body temperature is 37°C.)

Acute inflammation is generally only of short duration and can proceed to one of several conclusions:
1. It can successfully overcome the infection and the inflamed part is then repaired or replaced with scar tissue.
2. It can result in the formation of pus (suppuration).
3. It can extend, as when the organisms overcome the host's defences and the infection passes more deeply into the body involving tissue spaces, structures and organs and perhaps invading the bloodstream.
4. It can become chronic and persistent.

Suppuration. This occurs if the bacteria are able to kill some of the host's cells in the infected part. The inflammatory exudate is then full of living, dead and degenerating white cells together with living and dead organisms

63

and tissue cells and the resultant thick, creamy, opaque and sometimes bloodstained material is called *pus*.

Abscesses. An abscess is a collection of pus confined within the walls of a cavity formed by tissue degeneration. The essential local treatment of an abscess is to open it up to the surface and thus allow adequate drainage of the pus. This is achieved, for instance, in an apical dental abscess by opening the root canal or removing the infected tooth. When a deep abscess bursts through the overlying tissues to drain spontaneously on to the surface, the opening is called a *sinus*, e.g. the discharging sinus over the apex of a chronically infected tooth.

The general treatment of inflammation is aimed at maintaining the patient's strength, general health and resistance and reinforcing these when necessary with carefully chosen antibiotic drugs, e.g. penicillin, to which the causative organisms are known to be sensitive.

Cysts. A cyst is an abnormal cavity or sac within the body lined by well-defined epithelial and fibrous tissue and filled with a fluid or semi-solid material. Dental cysts are usually formed from a small cluster of epithelial cells deeply embedded in the tissues. As these cells multiply into a clump, the cells in the centre become deprived of nutrition from the surrounding blood supply and they degenerate and liquefy, while those at the outside continue to survive amd multiply. Fluid pressure increases inside the cavity as the products build up inside the wall of cells and a balloon-like expansion takes place.

Tumours. A tumour is a swelling, usually due to a new growth of cells (neoplasm) arising without known cause and growing without any relationship to normal growth, repair or health and thus serving no useful purpose. Tumours may be *benign* (localised and not invasive) or *malignant* (progressively invasive and growing at the expense of local tissue). Primarily malignant tumours can give rise to secondary 'seedling' tumours in other parts of the body when tiny fragments of the original tumour are carried in the lymphatics or bloodstream to other tissues or organs and start to grow there.

Ulcers. An ulcer is a localised lesion of the skin or mucous membrane where destruction of the surface epithelium exposes the deeper tissues in an open sore which may become secondarily infected. Ulcers may occur in the mouth that are due to a variety of causes, e.g. traumatic ulcers due to scratches or ill-fitting dentures, or herpetic ulcers as a result of a virus infection.

Diagnostic aids

Laboratory investigations for a patient are often an important aid to diagnosis and treatment planning. The taking, handling and transport of all these samples for diagnosis have to be carried out under strictly controlled aseptic conditions. This is (1) to protect the specimen and (2) to ensure that there is no danger of cross-infection.

Swabs. A swab can be taken of pus from an infected surface and then laboratory tests may be carried out to identify the pathogenic organism and discover the drugs to which it is sensitive so that appropriate treatment can be started.

Blood tests. A blood test can reveal important details about a patient such as his bleeding and clotting times, the number and types of blood cells present, the haemoglobin level, the blood group, the presence of infecting organisms and so on, as well as helping in the detection of specific diseases.

Biopsies. For a biopsy a small piece of diseased tissue is cut out of the lesion under examination and is then prepared, sectioned, stained and studied under the microscope. After this a detailed report can be made about the condition of the tissues and cells of the affected part.

DENTAL PATHOLOGY

Dental caries (Fig. 3/2)

This disease is a localised, post-eruptive, pathological process of external origin involving the softening and disintegration of the hard tooth tissues and proceeding to the formation of a cavity. It is the most universally prevalent disease afflicting the human race and is found particularly in people who live in civilised communities and eat a highly refined diet. The developmental pits and fissures are the first parts of the teeth to be affected and then the interproximal contact areas. In middle age, the necks of the teeth are more commonly at risk as the gingivae recede. At all stages local loss of tooth structure will allow the stagnation of food debris and possibly food packing between the teeth and damage to the gingival and periodontal structures.

Several theories have been put forward to explain the mechanisms responsible for the production of dental caries and the disease is the subject of constant research.

The most popular theory suggests that caries is due to the attack of acid-producing bacteria. Organisms can be found on the surfaces of the teeth having the ability to convert sugars and other fermentable carbohydrates to

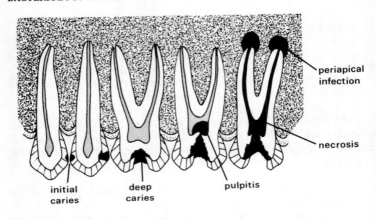

Fig. 3/2 The progress of untreated dental caries

lactic and other acids. When these organisms are allowed to collect undisturbed on the tooth surface, together with deposits of mucin from the saliva, epithelial cells and food debris, they quickly form a strongly adherent film called *dental plaque*. This deposit will occur most easily in areas that are not self-cleansing, e.g. pits and fissures and interdental spaces. These large numbers of organisms, protected from the acid-neutralising or buffering effects of saliva, can rapidly convert the sugary food debris and produce an acid strong enough to attack the enamel, and they will receive further supplies of sugars and fermentable carbohydrate in each mouthful that is put into the mouth. Gradually the surface of the enamel is decalcified and takes on a whitish appearance before it disintegrates allowing the organisms to invade the tooth. When the full depth of the enamel is involved, the process crosses the enamel-dentine (amelo-dentinal) junction and the inorganic part of the dentine is attacked and decalcified. This softened dentine, now directly open to the mouth, is soon invaded by protein-dissolving (proteolytic) organisms and the cavity rapidly enlarges, partly by extension along the enamel-dentine junction and partly by deeper penetration along the dentinal tubules towards the pulp. The pulp reacts by trying to wall off the approaching process by forming secondary dentine within the pulp chamber. Unless the carious process is arrested the pulp becomes inflamed and painful. Without treatment the pulp eventually dies, with relief of the pain, and the bacteria can then invade the pulp chamber. The infection may then pass through the apical foramen of the tooth and cause a peri-apical abscess. An acute peri-apical abscess causes pain and swelling of the alveolus ('gumboil') or of the facial tissues and lymph nodes in the region.

Periodontal disease (Fig. 3/3)

This is the general term used to describe abnormalities of the periodontium or supporting structures of the teeth (the cementum, the periodontal membrane, the alveolar bone and the overlying and investing tissues).

Inflammation of the gingival tissues (gingivitis) may arise from a variety of causes. The commonest local causes include soft foods that do nothing to stimulate and harden the gingival tissues; sharp, hard foods that scratch and damage the gingival tissues; inefficient tooth brushing and food debris stagnation; irregularly arranged teeth and traumatic bites; untreated dental caries or inadequate and badly contoured restorations; ill-fitting partial dentures or orthodontic appliances; and drying due to mouth breathing. Gingivitis is often associated with the formation of tartar (calculus) on the teeth. There may also be general factors involved such as vitamin deficiencies, blood disorders and drugs.

In chronic marginal gingivitis the gum margins are very slightly swollen and may bleed easily. If the disease is neglected the inflammation spreads deeper to involve the periodontal membrane, the gingivae become detached from the necks of the teeth and a pocket is formed in which further food debris and inflammatory products accumulate. This serious condition is usually painless and may pass unnoticed by the patient.

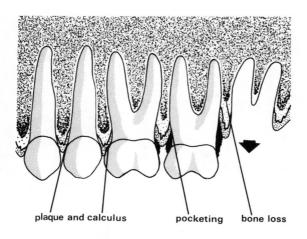

plaque and calculus   pocketing   bone loss

Fig. 3/3 The progress of untreated periodontal disease

Gradually, if still untreated, the gingival attachment recedes towards the apical region of the tooth, the pockets enlarge, the fibres of the periodontal membrane are progressively destroyed, the gingivae recede, the alveolar bone of the socket is resorbed and the tooth loosens.

Delay in discovering and treating this slow, insidious disease process will lead to the loss of many teeth, particularly in the over 35 age-group although the first stages of the disease can often be detected in adolescence.

Chapter Four

PRACTICE ORGANISATION

The majority of dental surgery assistants (DSAs) are employed in general practice, although they may also work in other clinical situations such as dental clinics, dental hospitals, dental departments of general hospitals and in specialist practices.

While this chapter describes in outline how the duties of the DSA fit into the organisation of general practice, it must be remembered that each individual practice has its own characteristics shaped by its situation and patients, size and internal layout and the dental surgeon's own personality and requirements.

The DSA must keep a flexible attitude of mind when she starts a new job in practice and be willing to learn about unfamiliar routines and working conditions before presuming to contribute suggestions based upon her own knowledge and experience.

The DSA becomes a key member of the dental health team, headed by the dental surgeon, which is devoted to the smooth, efficient running of the practice and to providing the highest standard of dental care for the patients. In small practices the DSA may be the only assistant the dental surgeon requires, but in large practices there will be more than one DSA and possibly a dental technician, a secretary/receptionist and an oral hygienist on the staff.

It is most important that the DSA maintains a professional relationship at all times with the patients, the dental surgeon and the other members of the dental team. She must not gossip about the privileged information she will gain within the practice; she must devote all her attention to the work of the practice while on duty; personal matters should be set aside to be dealt with outside surgery hours, e.g. the telephone must not be used for personal calls. Everything must be done to shield the dental surgeon from all unnecessary distractions so that he may concentrate all his time and attention upon the central and prime purpose of caring for his patients. In addition, skilled chairside assistance will mean that he will be able to work faster and more efficiently, thus making a greater contribution to the health of the community, as well as earning more money for the practice.

69

The rooms in general dental practice are usually allocated to serve different purposes as shown in Figure 4/1. In some practices a room can have more than one function, e.g. office/staff room or office/waiting room, while others may not have a laboratory or a dark room.

The duties of the trained DSA will include reception, surgery and secretarial work. Although in larger practices these duties may be shared between several members of the staff, the DSA must be capable of undertaking all these duties if required to do so.

RECEPTION

One of the most important aspects of a successful dental practice is the atmosphere surrounding the reception of patients and other callers on the telephone and at the door. This, the first contact that the perhaps nervous and apprehensive patient makes with the practice, will immediately set the tone of the whole encounter because it will be presumed to reflect the general interest and attitude of mind of the whole team.

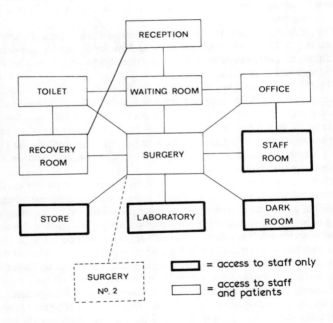

Fig. 4/1 Layout of rooms in a general dental practice

Telephone technique

1. All incoming calls should be answered as soon as possible.
2. Always smile while you speak on the telephone for this will give your voice a friendly, pleasant sound. You can remind yourself to smile by having a mirror in front of the telephone.
3. Answer the telephone efficiently by giving your own number and perhaps adding 'Mr Tooth's dental surgery – can I help you?' If you are very busy never say 'Hold on a minute!' and put down the receiver. Instead, ask the caller if he is prepared to wait or if he could call back in a few minutes, otherwise note the telephone number and arrange to call back later yourself.
4. Keep calls brief and to the point. Other patients may want to contact the practice also.
5. Take down any messages accurately and make sure that they reach their destination quickly. A message pad and pencil are essential next to the telephone.

Appointment book

The appointment book rules the speed at which a practice runs and the dental surgeon will indicate how much time he requires for each patient. Keep the book entries in pencil for easy alteration. Write in all appointments at the moment that they are made and always give the patient a written appointment card. Do not book long appointments so that they will overlap the lunch break. (Some dental surgeons will put fictitious names in the appointment book to allow necessary rest periods during the day.)

General reception

When patients arrive they are usually met by a member of the team and conducted to the waiting room. Make sure that everything is done to soothe their senses of sight, hearing and smell which may be enhanced by nervousness. All the rooms pertaining to the practice must be kept clean, bright and pleasant. All offensive odours including tobacco, the staff's lunchtime snacks, strong antiseptics, etc should be banned or dealt with by an aerosol air freshener.

The DSA must always have a neat, clean and tidy appearance, with a clean uniform, unobtrusive make-up and a neat hairstyle. Obviously she has well-cared-for teeth and good oral hygiene. She must balance speed and efficiency with professional charm, cheerfulness and sympathy when she greets a patient. Speed does not mean running about – 'a nurse only runs in the event of fire or haemorrhage'. She must remember that what for her is just another routine visit to the practice may represent a long-dreaded,

71

major event from the patient's point of view. People under stress may react in quite uncharacteristic ways, e.g. by becoming more talkative or quick to take offence or, at the other extreme, by becoming quieter and even tearful. Smiling, low-key, interested sympathy and 'time to listen' can help to soothe the patient from the start and reduce tensions in the surgery later. Try not to get involved with long descriptions of symptoms that will only have to be retold later to the dental surgeon. Never discuss details of treatment at this stage unless specifically instructed to do so by the dental surgeon.

Waiting room
In common with the rest, this room must be maintained in a clean, bright, warm and cheerful condition Sit in the waiting room yourself now and then and look around with a patient's eye. Are the chair springs broken? Is there dust under the table? Are the magazines dog-eared and out of date? Are the ash trays full? Are the mirrors smeared or dusty? and so on. Where security is good the patients should be encouraged to take off their coats and hats and leave them in the waiting room so that time is not wasted in the surgery.

DUTIES OF THE DENTAL SURGERY ASSISTANT (DSA)

In general the DSA's duties in the dental surgery are concerned with:

Maintenance of equipment. To maintain the equipment, instruments and furnishings in good working order and in a high state of cleanliness and preparation. This can be done efficiently if special check lists are made out to indicate a schedule of daily, weekly, monthly and half-yearly tasks which will include everything from switching the equipment on in the morning, oiling the handpieces, cleaning out the spittoon traps, draining the air compressor, polishing and cleaning the surfaces in the surgery right through to arranging a regular visit by the maintenance engineer from the dental company's service department. Check lists mean that you do not have to rely on your memory.

Expendable items. To ensure that adequate stocks of expendable drugs, materials and instruments are immediately available. Make frequent stock list checks with your dental surgeon. Always keep available a spare operating light bulb and fuses for the dental unit. Know where tools such as a screwdriver are kept.

Patients' records. To ensure that all the relevant dental records, radiographs, appliances and models are immediately available for all patients visiting the surgery on that day. This usually means that they have to be got out of the files the day before. It is helpful to keep a list of the day's appointments in the surgery and at reception.

Preparation of patients for treatment. To assist patients into the surgery and get them settled in the chair and prepared for treatment with the minimum of delay, e.g. ladies should be given a tissue to remove their lipstick.

Assistance during treatment. To produce instruments and materials as necessary during treatment, quickly and efficiently and to assist the dental surgeon as he requests it. The extent to which the DSA is expected to help in this respect will vary from one dental surgeon to another and will depend also upon the design of the surgery. It usually involves suction, retraction, manipulation of the air and water syringes, changing burs in the handpiece, passing instruments and mixing and passing materials.

Making the next appointment. To assist the patient from the surgery without unnecessary delay and arranging for the next appointment to be made.

Treatment record. To make sure that an adequate written record is kept of all treatment provided.

Cleaning up. To tidy up between patients, clean and sterilise the instruments and remove all traces of the visit.

Awareness of special patient problems. Although every patient attending the dental surgery must be granted full attention and care at all times, certain categories of patient present special problems that require extra thought and preparation. These are usually patients suffering from a particular disability or handicap. Such disabilities are commonly classified as follows: *medical*, e.g. the asthmatic patient or the patient who is recovering from a heart condition and taking drugs to prevent further blood clots occurring; *physical*, e.g. the blind or paralysed patient; *mental*, e.g. the patient with Down's syndrome (mongolism), or the retarded patient, and *social*, e.g. the child from a broken home. The extent of special care for such patients may even require the dental surgeon and the DSA to make a domiciliary visit to carry out dental treatment in the patient's own home.

SURGERY DESIGN

There are many different working arrangements but they generally fall into one of the following categories:

The dental surgeon works standing up. All equipment and cabinets are fixed, but within easy reach a step or two away from the chair. A single dental unit will suffice. The DSA assists from the patient's left side when required.

The dental surgeon is seated. This means that he is no longer mobile and all equipment has to be brought nearer to the chair for him to reach it, or else handed to him. The DSA must spend more time at the chairside, but will have to have access to equipment on both sides of the chair during treatment.

Four-handed dentistry. The dental surgeon and the DSA are both seated. All equipment is within easy reach of both of them, or the DSA only, and can be passed freely to and fro. This is a less tiring arrangement and means that four hands are available to carry out treatment in the patient's mouth. It may take a few weeks for the close teamwork required to be achieved but once gained, the speed of treatment to a high standard is greatly enhanced. Low-level stools will require low-level working surfaces and a dental chair without too many levers, etc projecting in the way of the team's knees. The DSA may move away from the chairside for other duties such as sterilising instruments.

Six-handed dentistry. The dental surgeon and the DSA are both seated as before, but to minimise their time away from the chairside, a second DSA is always available to sterilise and replenish instruments, prepare materials and generally work in support of the other two. There should be frequent interchange of the two DSAs to ensure that they are both fully trained in chairside duties and thus avoid the dental surgeon becoming totally dependent on one assistant with unsettling results to the practice in the event of holidays, illness and so on.

Surgery equipment
The following items will be found in most dental surgeries:

A dental unit. This contains and supports such things as the operating light, air-spray, water-spray, suction and saliva ejector, the dental engine, air-rotor or air-motor, a spittoon and a sterilisable working surface or bracket table. The unit may be a single pedestal or split into two sections one on each side of the chair.

A dental chair. Most dental surgeons now operate with the patient lying in the supine position; high-speed suction becomes essential to protect the patient's airway. The dental chair has a mechanism (sometimes programmed) for raising, lowering and tilting it until the patient's mouth is at a convenient working height for the dental surgeon. In some circumstances the patient has to be treated sitting up, e.g. if suffering from an arthritic condition, and most modern dental chairs can be adjusted to accommodate these requirements.

Cabinets and trolleys. These are best grouped as close as possible to the working area so that instruments, materials and working surfaces are conveniently to hand during treatment procedures.

Operating stools. When the dental team can sit down to work they will be less tired at the end of the day. Positioning is very important, otherwise the DSA may get into the bad habit of working in a crouched, unbalanced position that can be just as tiring as working standing up. Try to sit upright with both feet comfortably flat on the floor and the spine and neck straight and upright. Working surfaces and the patient's mouth height should ideally be at elbow height so that the hands and forearms are working in the least tiring position.

Sterilising apparatus. Unless a sterile package or tray system is used, this apparatus must be switched on at the earliest opportunity in the day so that it is fully heated up and ready for action at the start of the treatment session. Some instruments are sterilised afresh each day and then stored in covered trays of antiseptic solution all day ready for immediate use.

X-ray apparatus. This generally requires little attention apart from cleaning and dusting the outer surfaces. The apparatus should be switched off at the main electric source when not in use. (Keep a careful eye on the condition of the exposed wiring, for these machines develop high voltages.)

Hand instruments. These must be maintained at a very high standard and checked frequently. Moving parts must be oiled regularly, e.g. handpieces. Sharpening chisels and excavators can only be learned by watching a practical demonstration. They can be ruined by inexpert sharpening and some dental surgeons prefer to sharpen hand instruments themselves.

Dental materials. These form an expensive item in any practice budget and should be used economically. Although replacement stocks must be available it is obviously ill-advised to order large quantities of materials which may deteriorate before they are used. Under normal conditions the DSA will not be expected to order any stocks without first consulting the dental surgeon about it.

The scrap residues of certain materials such as amalgam, mercury, gold and the lead foil from x-ray packages are valuable and should be saved up as they are saleable.

Some disposable items may be dangerous if they fall into wrong hands and should be totally destroyed before being placed in waste bins, e.g. hypodermic needles, disposable syringes. Remains of drugs, e.g. the contents of half-used cartridges of local anaesthetic, should be washed away down the sink. Discarded sharp instruments, e.g. scalpel blades, are potentially dangerous and must be disposed of with care.

Specialist apparatus. There may be many other pieces of apparatus present in the surgery, e.g. anaesthetic machines, spot-welders, ultrasonic scalers and so on, that will require special care and maintenance. The DSA should find out what unfamiliar apparatus is for, how it works and whether she is responsible for its maintenance. Some types of specialist apparatus are easily and expensively damaged by the untaught.

Emergency equipment. Make sure that you know where the surgical emergency equipment is kept and that it is always in good order. If any part of it is used at any time make sure that it is replaced immediately. See also Recovery Room below.

THE RECOVERY ROOM

This is used for patients who need to lie down for a while to recover from a general anaesthetic or from a reaction to treatment, such as fainting, before they are fit to leave for home.

Equipment
The equipment in a recovery room will usually consist of:
    A firm couch and pillows with washable covers
    A supply of blankets
    A good light source at the patient's head for observing his colour and to
        illuminate any intra-oral procedures
    Bowls for vomit, blood and mouthwashing
    A supply of towels, preferably disposable
    Mouthwash cups
    A mirror for the patients to tidy their appearance afterwards.

Emergency equipment
Emergency equipment and services may be duplicated here and in the surgery, e.g. suction, oxygen, gags, airways, cardiac and respiratory stimulant drugs, syringes and hypodermic needles, sterile artery forceps, gauze packs. In general practice this room may only be used at infrequent

intervals, but it must be maintained in constant readiness and its contents and cleanliness should be added to the weekly check list apart from the immediate cleaning that is required each time it is used.

DARK ROOM

This is where dental radiographs are processed and is used on all occasions when light-sensitive film has to be handled.

Essential features
These are:
    Light-proof window covers
    Photographic safe-lights and independent ordinary lights
    A door-locking system so designed that there is no danger of accidental
        admission of light during film processing
    Developing, washing and fixing tanks and a source of running water
    Electric tank heaters and a thermometer
    A clock with an alarm timing system
    X-ray film hangers, films, cassettes and a store of chemicals
    A place to hang processed films to dry
    A container for scrap foil and a bin for waste paper
    An adequate ventilation system to eliminate chemical fumes.

This room has to be kept clean and dust-free. Splashes of chemical solutions must be wiped up immediately. All solutions must be maintained as indicated in the manufacturers' instructions. *Note*. X-ray films can also be processed in daylight using special light-proof developing tanks and apparatus such as the Kodak 'Dentech' processor.

DENTAL LABORATORY

This is rarely in the DSA's province, but she needs to know where things are kept, particularly impressions, models and completed work. The liaison between the DSA and the laboratory technicians must be maintained at a friendly, mutually helpful level so that the work flows smoothly and adequate time is given for each laboratory stage to be completed. In all cases requiring laboratory work always consult the technician before arranging the patient's next appointment. Make sure that the work-slip is clearly made out. If possible arrange for the work to be ready at the start of the morning or afternoon session so that the dental surgeon has time to examine it before the patient arrives. In some practices work is sent out to a laboratory and great care must be taken to pack fragile models and wax-ups with plenty of padding so that they are not damaged in transit. Some dental surgeons will teach their DSA to cast up impressions as soon as they are taken to avoid possible distortion or breakages if casting is delayed.

OFFICE

The DSA's duties and responsibilities in the office will vary from practice to practice. In some cases a special secretary is employed to run the office, while in other, smaller practices the DSA will be expected to carry out most of this work herself, under the supervision of the dental surgeon. The following lists briefly indicate some of the more important aspects of office work, but must not be regarded as comprehensive. The range of work may seem formidable, but it can be reduced to an easily controllable amount by a tidy, systematic approach. The future of office administration will obviously be affected by the rapidly expanding usage of microprocessors in the handling of information both in the form of figures and words and it may be assumed that the DSA will shortly be involved in this (Fig. 4/2).

Current microprocessors consist basically of a keyboard, similar to that of a typewriter, a visual display unit (VDU) resembling a standard television screen, together with methods of electrically recording information on discs or tapes and a print-out mechanism which itself can type like a

Fig. 4/2 A microprocessor system that can be used to handle information and records in dental practice

typewriter. This apparatus can be used to store information such as address lists, details of patients' treatments, waiting lists, recall lists, stock control, accounting and tax details, and can recall and display or print-out such information instantly. The information can be up-dated easily, and the storage space required is much less than that for similar information on paper. The future uses of such apparatus appear to be limitless.

Office equipment

Desk or work table	Telephone
Chairs	Typewriter
Good light source	Waste-paper basket
Filing cabinets or	General reference books
cupboards, safe or cash box	

Office stocks

Headed notepaper	Receipt forms or book
Plain typing paper,	Appointment cards
top and copy qualities	Recall cards
Envelopes	Laboratory slips
Treatment record cards for	Message pads
new patients: NHS and Private	Carbon paper
X-ray envelopes	Spare typewriter ribbon
NHS forms, envelopes, etc	Writing materials: pens,
Anaesthetic consent forms	pencils, erasers, paper clips, etc
Bill forms	Postage stamps

Professional records

Patients' records and radiographs, filed as follows:
  NHS
  Private
  On treatment
  Off treatment
  Awaiting payment
Patients' correspondence—doctors, dental surgeons, hospitals, NHS, etc
Appointment book
Day book (records the fee earned immediately each patient leaves the surgery)
Recall lists
Models (under 200 models can be stored alphabetically, over 200 should be stored numerically and an index book used)

Financial records
General accounts:
  General account book
  Petty cash book
  Wages book
  Bills and receipts of practice expenses
Patients' accounts:
  Accounts for treatment completed/dates presented and paid
  Day book, as mentioned above
Banking matters:
  Bank statements, paying-in book, the practice cheque book
  All these records have to be produced for the accountant annually for
  him to prepare a general statement of the affairs of the practice and deal
  with taxation matters
Tax matters:
  Demands, letters, receipts
Postage book (records of postage stamps used and posting dates)

General information
Surgery routine check lists
Information book, which lists such things as the names, addresses and
  telephone numbers of: accountant; anaesthetist; electrician; equipment
  servicing agents; dental companies; plumber; special dental
  laboratories; laundry; printers, and so on
Stores lists with dates orders made and received
Drug lists
Poisons records
Accident record book
Precious metals record
Laundry book or lists
Practice documents:
  Instruction leaflets
  Hire purchase agreements
  Insurance policies, etc
Holiday lists
Records of instruments being repaired or taken out of the practice for use
  elsewhere, e.g. in an operating theatre

Chapter Five

STERILISATION AND ASEPSIS

All dental treatment must be carried out under conditions which will reduce the dangers of cross-infection by the transmission of pathogenic micro-organisms both to and from the patient. Such contamination may occur via the surroundings, instruments, materials or the dental team themselves. The DSA must remain alert to this ever-present hazard at all times, for everyone's health and safety in the dental surgery depend upon her constant and meticulous care in these matters.

STERILISATION

Sterilisation is a most important factor in the prevention of cross-infection. Sterile means completely free from all forms of life. Sterilisation is the production of sterility by the complete removal or destruction of living micro-organisms and their spores from instruments and other material and may be achieved by heat, chemical or irradiation methods.

Central sterile supply department (CSSD)
Large hospitals use the CSSD system in which all used equipment is returned to one department for disposal or to be cleaned and sterilised before re-issue. By concentrating all this work in one place the risk of cross-infection is reduced. The system requires duplication of many instruments and is thus too expensive for routine dental practice.

Cleaning instruments, prior to sterilisation
Before sterilisation, used instruments should be scrubbed clean with soap and water, and then rinsed, for any debris may act as a barrier to the sterilising process. It is strongly advised that the DSA should herself wear thick rubber gloves when she undertakes this preliminary process to protect herself from accidental infection from the dirty instruments. When the debris is firmly attached, e.g. dried blood, thorough cleaning can be achieved with an ultrasonic cleaner. Instruments are placed in a bath of

STERILISATION AND ASEPSIS

detergent solution and subjected to high-frequency vibration which breaks up and shakes off even minute particles, very thoroughly, in a few minutes. The detergent must be rinsed off before sterilisation.

Sterilisation by moist heat

Boiling water. When instruments and utensils are boiled in water (100°C) for 15 minutes most pathogenic organisms are killed, but this method cannot destroy some highly resistant spores of certain viruses, e.g. the hepatitis virus which causes a highly infectious and dangerous disease. Thus boiling water is said to disinfect but **not** sterilise. It is mentioned here because it was once the traditional method used everywhere, but now it must be regarded as an emergency measure to be used only when alternative methods are not available.

Autoclave. This is the most reliable method of sterilising instruments, utensils and other equipment in the dental surgery. Water boils at 100°C at normal atmospheric pressure. If the water is heated in a closed container, such as an autoclave, the steam pressure and the temperature continue to rise as the system is heated until at a pressure of 2.2 bar (32 lbs per square inch) the temperature reaches 134°C. No living thing can survive after three minutes' exposure to steam at this temperature.

Steam under pressure can penetrate porous substances, but not air-tight containers. The items to be sterilised are placed in perforated metal containers or drums or may be loosely wrapped in special paper or paper bags. Steam corrosion of certain instruments after autoclaving can be prevented by wrapping them in paper impregnated with vapour-phase inhibitor. Paper wrappings and containers are sealed with heat-sensitive adhesive tape which changes colour when heated, thus distinguishing between treated and untreated packages.

The small autoclave works by electricity. The apparatus has to be 'topped-up' with distilled water to the required level each morning. Before opening the door of the autoclave check that the pressure gauge registers zero. The door is then opened and the prepared packages and containers are loaded into the autoclave, taking care to allow sufficient space for steam to circulate between them (Fig. 5/1). The door is closed firmly , the locking mechanism engaged and the starting button or switch operated to set the automatic cycle in motion. The pressure will rise gradually, slowly if this is the first load of the day, but more rapidly when the apparatus has been pre-heated by previous operating cycles. The pressure should reach 2.2 bar at which time the thermometer should register 134°C and the timer should enable this condition to be maintained for well over the required three minutes. Finally the cycle is completed by the automatic release of the steam pressure, with the condensation of the steam back into water and a

82

reduction of pressure. The door may then be opened safely and the still hot containers and packets removed with an asbestos glove or special forceps. The open steam-circulation ports on autoclave drums should be closed to prevent contamination from the air. Large hospital and commercial autoclaves of the *downward displacement* or *high vacuum* types use chambers, from which air can be exhausted (heated by dry steam from an external source).

The efficiency of the autoclave process can be checked by including with the load an indicator or 'teller' which shows a change when the required temperature is reached, e.g. Browne's Steriliser Control Tubes, which are sealed glass tubes containing an indicator solution that changes from red through amber to green upon reaching the temperature they have been designed for.

Items that have been sterilised in this way may be stored in dry, dust-free conditions in the dental surgery and the containers or packets opened as required at a later date. Items wrapped in paper should be used within three days or else re-sterilised. Sterile cheatle forceps should be used to remove dressings, etc from the interior of sterile drums which should be closed again immediately.

Fig. 5/1 Instruments being placed into a small steam autoclave prior to the sterilisation cycle

Sterilisation by dry heat

Hot-air oven. Cleaned, heat-resistant equipment can be sterilised by subjecting it to hot air at a temperature of 160°C for one hour. Electrically heated hot-air oven sterilisers have a thermometer, a thermostat and a timing switch so that they can be set to operate under the required conditions.

Instruments are generally put into tape-sealed metal containers before being placed in the oven. The load must be loosely packed to allow circulation of air. Hot air is very useful for sterilising sharp instruments and root canal therapy boxes, though in the latter, paper points and cotton-wool may be discoloured by the heat. The load should be allowed to cool before it is removed from the oven to avoid contaminated air being drawn into contracting packages.

Hot oils. In this method oil is heated to a temperature of 100°C or above and the instruments are placed in it for periods of about ten minutes. It has been suggested that this technique is suitable for handpieces and other instruments with working parts. It cannot, however, be recommended because of the poor penetration of the hot oil and also its doubtful effectiveness in killing spores.

Molten metal, etc. Electrically-heated containers are available which hold and heat up small quantities of molten metal, salt or glass beads to over 200°C. During root canal therapy small instruments and paper points held in tweezers may be dipped repeatedly into the heated material for 5 to 15 seconds to re-sterilise their surfaces during treatment and thus help to disinfect the root canal. They have very limited application and are a source of danger if overturned.

Flaming with alcohol. This out-of-date and dangerous method of disinfection is mentioned here only to condemn it. Alcohol is wiped over a heat-resistant surface, e.g. the inside of a metal kidney dish, and then ignited. But the layer of unburnt alcohol vapour between the surface and the flame prevents the surface from being heated effectively.

Direct heat. Metal can be sterilised by heating it in a flame until it is red hot. This method is used in bacteriological investigations where a platinum wire loop is used to transfer infected material, e.g. pus, from one place to another. Such a wire loop is sterilised by holding it in a gas flame. Dental instruments would be ruined if heated in this way.

Sterilisation by chemicals

Most germicidal chemicals, with the exception of the gases described below, are unsuitable for the purpose of sterilisation. They have limited application and many spores and viruses are highly resistant to them for long periods. Sterilisation by chemical solutions (generally only suitable for clean, hard, resistant surfaces) is now largely superseded by physical sterilisation methods in general dental surgery.

Solutions. Some previously sterilised instruments may be stored for short periods by immersing them in antiseptic or disinfectant solutions, e.g. alcohol 70%; Roccal 1:1000; phenol 1:40; contained in a sterile dish with a suitable lid. Certain items that would be damaged by heat sterilisation methods can be sterilised by immersion for 10 minutes in a 2% activitated glutaraldehyde solution. Strong disinfectant solutions must be rinsed away with sterile water before the instrument is used to avoid chemical burns to the tissues.

Gases. Certain equipment may be sterilised by exposing it to gases or vapours in a closed container. This method can be used in industry but is unsuitable for dental practice. The gases are:
(a) Formaldehyde vapour, which has a poor capacity for penetration and a very slow sterilising action
(b) Ethylene oxide gas, which is expensive, has a limited application and is highly explosive.

Sterilisation by irradiation
Ionising gamma radiation. This physical method is commonly used in industry to sterilise a wide range of disposable materials and equipment that is obtainable in sealed packages and containers. A large, elaborate sterilising plant is required with adequate safety precautions. The gamma radiation is obtained from radioactive sources such as Cobalt 60. The rays can penetrate most materials and kill all organisms and spores very quickly. Disposable gloves, plastic surgical equipment, syringes, needles, suture materials, dressings, plasma, drugs destroyed by heat and so on may all be sterilised in this way.

Some particular problems of sterilisation
Handpieces. In general, all handpieces can be sterilised in the autoclave (134°C) provided that the following special precautions are taken. They must first be thoroughly cleaned in the manner recommended by the manufacturer. It has been shown that lubricating oil remaining within the handpiece shields protects the spores of many organisms from the pressurised steam. This problem is overcome when the instrument has been treated by spraying a special penetrating additive into the retained oil which then vapourises in the autoclave and destroys the organisms.

Handpieces so treated are inserted into sealed containers or sachets before being placed in the autoclave so that they can be stored in a sterile condition until required. Handpieces can also be sterilised in a hot oven but the DSA should always check the manufacturer's instructions.

Air turbines. These can be sterilised in the autoclave after first removing the plastic bur chuck, and preferably after the above mentioned penetrating additive treatment. They must *not* be placed in the hot air oven because they will be damaged by the high temperature.

Rubber gloves. These are generally disposable, but they may be re-sterilised in the autoclave in a cotton envelope or wallet. A small quantity of special glove powder is sterilised at the same time. Gloves should be washed, examined for punctures and the cuffs folded back several inches before placing them in the wallet.

Glassware. This must be thoroughly cleaned with a detergent, rinsed and sterilised in the autoclave.

Glass clinical thermometers. These cannot be heated, but should be rinsed thoroughly in cold water and placed in a disinfectant solution. This solution should be changed frequently to ensure its effectiveness, and always rinsed off before the thermometer is used again. Alternatively, they may be disinfected in 70% alcohol and stored dry.

Plastics. Equipment made of polyvinyl chloride (PVC), polytetra-fluorethylene (PTFE) and polyethylene can be sterilised by autoclaving. New equipment should be boiled first in several changes of distilled water to remove any water-soluble traces in the plastic.

Polystyrene will melt at autoclave temperatures and can only be effectively sterilised with gamma rays or ethylene oxide gas. Acrylic (Perspex) is damaged by heat and gamma rays. Most chemical disinfectant solutions are absorbed by or damage heat-moulded plastics in the long run.

Rubber. Such equipment may be sterilised by autoclaving. New natural or silicone rubber apparatus should be boiled first in several changes of distilled water, as with plastics.

ASEPSIS

Asepsis is achieved when all living disease-causing micro-organisms have been killed or removed from the equipment in use and the immediate environment of the patient.

Dental procedures can be considered to be of two kinds:

Surgical operations

In these the outer defensive tissues of the body are penetrated and the resultant wound is open to infection, e.g. dental extraction, injection, root canal therapy. Any procedure that involves entry into the blood- and serum-carrying tissues falls into this category. During all surgical procedures a strictly *aseptic technique* is essential and only sterile equipment may come into contact with the wound and its surrounding parts.

Non-surgical or routine treatment

The procedures in these cases do not penetrate the soft tissues, e.g. impressions, simple conservation treatment, topical applications. During non-surgical treatment the normal routines of cleanliness and general hygiene must be observed to prevent cross-infection (to other patients and members of the dental team), but the strict aseptic techniques are not required.

ASEPTIC TECHNIQUES

Environment

Air. Everything must be done to reduce air-borne contamination. The surgery should be as dust-free as possible. The ventilation and heating should be planned to help in this respect. Ideally, surgery should be carried out in a special room set aside for that purpose and casual visitors forbidden, to prevent additional dust and organisms being brought in on their clothes, shoes, hair, skin and from the upper respiratory tract, etc. In an operating theatre the staff don special theatre boots and clean linen theatre clothes before entering the surgical areas.

Furniture and equipment. The walls and ceiling should be cleaned frequently and the floor washed daily with a disinfectant solution. All dust-collecting sufaces should be washed frequently, ideally every day. The handbasin, taps and drains should be treated with disinfectant daily. General cleaning should be completed at least an hour before surgery to allow any remaining dust to settle. All metal and glass surfaces of dental equipment must be wiped over with a disinfecting solution between patients.

The dental team

Under ideal surgical conditions, in an operating theatre, both the dental surgeon and his assistant should wear a mask and cap, special clean theatre boots or overshoes, waterproof apron, 'scrub up' their hands and don a sterile gown and rubber gloves before the operation begins. The extent to which this extreme standard of theatre dress is observed in the dental surgery will depend upon the decision of the individual dental surgeon and the type of operation being undertaken. Its absence must not be taken as a signal to relax the other rigid standards that are required to maintain the aseptic technique vital to safe surgery.

Mask. This may be of disposable paper, synthetic fibre or cloth. Masks are worn by the operating team to reduce the danger of infection from their mouths and upper respiratory tracts contaminating the wound. They are not perfect guards, for some micro-organisms can still pass through them. The operator and assistants should cover all cuts and abrasions on their own faces with waterproof dressings. The mask should be put into position before scrubbing the hands and not touched again until the operation is completed.

Cap. This must be worn so as to cover the hair completely and prevent organisms falling on to the wound from that source. The cap also should be put on before the hands are scrubbed.

Apron. When ordinary everyday clothes are worn in the theatre it is best to cover them with a waterproof apron, otherwise if the sterile gown is subsequently wetted with water or blood, this will soak through and the gown will become contaminated by the non-sterile clothing underneath.

Hands. The skin of the hands harbours many pathogenic micro-organisms and it cannot be sterilised. However well the surface of the skin is cleaned, perspiration brings hordes of new organisms to the surface from the depths of the sweat glands.

The hands should be well cared for at all times, with short nails and a healthy, unbroken skin. Any cuts or abrasions of the hands should be covered with waterproof adhesive plaster. 'Scrubbing-up' before an operation entails scrubbing the fingernails with a sterile brush for one minute and then washing the hands and forearms for three minutes using antiseptic soap and a constant stream of warm water. Using special antiseptic soaps, e.g. 3% hexachlorophane, means that after the initial scrub for the first case on an operating list, the hands may be adequately cleaned by just washing them with soap and water for subsequent cases.

The hands are rinsed free of soap, keeping them raised above elbow level, and the taps turned off with the elbow, for now that the hands are clean they must not be contaminated by water from higher up the arms or contact with non-sterile surfaces. The hands, and then the arms, are dried carefully with a sterile towel or rinsed in 70% alcohol and allowed to dry completely in air.

Gown. The sterile operating gown is opened up carefully at arms' length taking care not to touch or contaminate the outside surfaces. The arms are slipped up into the sleeves and an assistant ties the neck tapes. The waist tapes should be held out sideways by their extreme ends so that an assistant can take them easily and tie them behind the waist.

Gloves. Rubber gloves, of various sizes, are provided in sterile wallets together with a packet of glove powder. The wallet is opened carefully, the powder packet extracted and its talc-like contents dusted over the hands and between the fingers. A small amount of powder may also be dusted into the interior of the gloves. One glove is removed from the wallet, holding it by its folded-back cuff, so that only the *inside* of the glove is touched by the skin, and slipped on to the hand. The second glove is now removed by slipping the fingers of the gloved hand underneath the folded-back cuff so that only the *outside* of the second glove is touched by the first. The second hand is inserted into the glove. Finally the cuffs of the gloves are unfolded back to cover and grip the gown sleeves, making sure that the gloved fingers only come into contact with the *outside* of the sterile gloves and are not contaminated from the skin surfaces.

Having reached this stage the members of the operating team must not touch a non-sterile surface or object (apart from the operation site) for if they do they must retire from the scene of the operation and carry out the 'scrubbing-up' process again.

Instruments and materials

Sterile instruments and materials must be set out by the 'no touch' technique which can only be learnt by actual practice. An 'unscrubbed' assistant can manipulate sterile towels and equipment using long-handled sterile cheatle forceps. Clean tables and trolleys may be set out by first covering them with a sterile waterproof sheet then a sterile towel and then placing sterile instruments, dressings and containers, e.g. gallipots and kidney dishes, on the towel as required. Sterile drums may be opened by hand, but their contents must only be touched with sterile forceps. Sealed paper packages of instruments may be torn open at one end and their contents slid out, untouched, on to the sterile towel or into a sterile dish. A laid-up trolley may be further protected until it is required by covering it with another sterile towel.

The patient

In the operating theatre the patient is draped with sterile waterproof sheeting covered with sterile towels held in place with sterile towel clips so that only the operation site, the mouth, is left exposed. The skin around the mouth and the oral mucosa may be cleaned with non-irritant antiseptic solutions.

In the dental surgery the patient's outdoor clothing and hair may be covered in a similar way. In the conscious patient saliva flowing near the operation site may be kept clear with adequate suction through a sterile sucker tip (Fig. 5/2). Wounds must *never* be irrigated with water from the dental unit sprays but only with sterile water or saline delivered by sterilised syringe or drip system.

Special precautions

Certain diseases, e.g. viral hepatitis (an infection of the liver tissue), are of particular interest and danger to the dental profession because they are highly contagious and can be transmitted by minute amounts of infected blood or saliva. Thus the dental team and future patients in the surgery are at risk from such things as droplet infection from air-rotor aerosols, infected instruments and other apparatus, and any other items that have become contaminated. The normal processes of meticulous sterilisation should suffice to protect everyone – in most cases. However, in recent years a particular hazard has been identified with regard to patients who have, or who are acting as carriers of, infection from a specific virus causing hepatitis – hepatitis B virus. This virus is particularly virulent and causes a

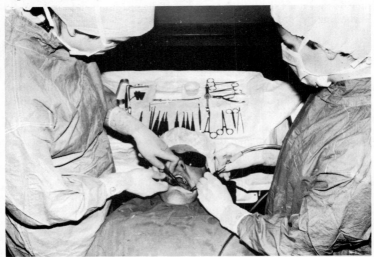

Fig. 5/2 An oral surgery procedure under strictly aseptic conditions. The DSA is maintaining good visibility using a narrow suction tip to draw off blood and irrigating saline, and by retracting tissues as directed by the operator

severe illness. It is recommended that when treatment of a known carrier of hepatitis B virus (or any other infective disease) is undertaken the following precautions, in addition to those already described for routine sterilisation, should be observed:

1. Wear rubber gloves and a gown and use an aseptic technique.
2. Wear a face mask together with spectacles or an eyeshield.
3. Use as many disposable instruments and dressings as possible; after treatment put all used disposable items and needles in an impervious container and incinerate them.
4. Disinfect all working surfaces and equipment controls after use.
5. Treat known carriers at the *end* of a session.
6. Avoid using the air-rotor, or ultrasonic scalers, to reduce aerosols.
7. Impressions should be treated by immersing them in special sterilising solutions (these will depend upon the type of impression material being used) before sending them to the laboratory.
8. Hands should be washed again after removing gown and gloves. Any area of skin that might be contaminated by blood must immediately be washed thoroughly. Any puncture wounds must be encouraged to bleed freely and then washed with soap and water.

If, in spite of these precautions, any member of the team should become exposed to infection, it is most important to seek immediate medical advice.

AIDS (Acquired immune deficiency syndrome)

The full disease process is not yet thoroughly understood, but it may be due to an infectious agent, probably a virus (HTLV III). It appears that the disease is transmitted via the body fluids particularly semen, blood and plasma products. At present the majority of cases are found in male homosexuals, but cases have been reported in women and children. AIDS leaves the patient vulnerable to opportunistic diseases which in turn may result in specific lung infections, fungal, bacterial and virus infections and certain cancers, e.g. Kaposi's sarcoma. Information that a patient suffers from AIDS or is an HTLV III carrier must be regarded as strictly confidential. Identified AIDS patients requiring dental treatment need to be cared for from a basis of sympathetic understanding; although it appears to be unlikely that alerted health care personnel will contract the disease from these patients every precaution to protect the members of the team and other patients must be observed.

It is recommended that known carriers of hepatitis B or HTLV III viruses and patients suffering from AIDS, should be treated in hospital dental departments that have appropriate facilities.

Chapter Six

DENTAL RECORDS AND CHARTING

THE DENTAL RECORD

Case history taking, clinical examination, diagnostic tests and treatment planning together form the foundation of all successful dental care. Accurate and up-to-date records of every stage of examination and treatment are essential to ensure continuity of treatment and to protect the dental surgeon in the unlikely event of legal proceedings by a dissatisfied patient. Most dental surgeons follow a methodical system such as:

Name
Age
Address and Telephone Number
Occupation
Name and Address of General Medical Practitioner
PMH (Previous Medical History)
PDH (Previous Dental History)
C/O (Patient Complains Of . . .)
O/E (On Examination)
  Extra-Oral
  Intra-Oral (includes making a chart of the teeth)
Provisional Diagnosis
  Special Tests (to investigate further)
Firm Diagnosis
Treatment Plan (immediate and long-term)

The DSA must be prepared to write down all these details as they are dictated to her by the dental surgeon, unless he prefers to make this record himself.

The dental chart

This is the most important record of the patient's dental condition. Usually the dental surgeon calls out the teeth, stating the cavities, fillings and so on as he discovers them during his intra-oral examination and the DSA makes an accurate representation of the presence and condition of the teeth by filling in symbols and outlines on a standard chart of the mouth (Figs. 6/1 and 6/2).

Fig. 6/1 Teeth chart

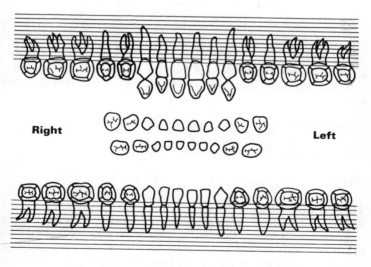

Fig. 6/2 Anatomical chart for periodontal records

The 32 permanent teeth and the 20 primary teeth can be described in words or numerical symbols.

The quadrant system
In this commonly used system, the mouth is divided into four segments and the teeth are designated as follows:

Permanent Teeth

Primary Teeth

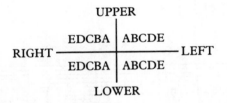

It should be noted that 'Right' and 'Left' are the patient's right and left.

In this way individual teeth can be described as in the following examples:

'Upper right five' = $\underline{5}|$ = upper right second premolar

'Lower left one' = $|\overline{1}$ = lower left central incisor

'Upper left C' = $|\underline{C}$ = upper left primary canine

The two-digit system
This international system for designating teeth is used by some dental surgeons, mostly outside Great Britain, because it simplifies the handling and communication of dental data, for example in computer programming. The quadrants are allocated digits 1 to 4 for permanent teeth in a clockwise sequence on the chart starting at the right upper side:

Permanent Teeth

	Upper Right			Upper Left	

Upper Right
18 17 16 15 14 13 12 11
48 47 46 45 44 43 42 41
Lower Right

Upper Left
21 22 23 24 25 26 27 28
31 32 33 34 35 36 37 38
Lower Left

Primary Teeth

Upper Right
55 54 53 52 51
85 84 83 82 81
Lower Right

Upper Left
61 62 63 64 65
71 72 73 74 75
Lower Left

Examples:
'One-two'   = 12 = upper right second incisor
'Three-eight' = 38 = lower left third molar
'Five-four'   = 54 = upper right first primary molar

The surfaces of the teeth. These are described by their anatomical names. Sometimes the words describing the surfaces involved in a cavity are abbreviated to their initial letters, e.g. mesio-occluso-distal, disto-occlusal or occluso-buccal become MOD, DO or OB.

The standard charts are usually diagrammatic (Fig. 6/1) but occasionally the crowns of the teeth are anatomically represented. Other charts are available for specialised purposes. In periodontal treatment a representation of the roots of the teeth will be necessary to record the depths of any pockets around the teeth (Fig. 6/2). In cases of fracture of the jaws a representation of the whole skull will enable the surgeon to keep an accurate record of gross bony injuries.

Common charting symbols
Tooth present and sound   ·
Tooth unerupted   u
Tooth missing   —
Tooth to be extracted   /
Tooth recently extracted   ×
Root present   +
Cavity   ○
Filling   ●
Unsound filling present to be restored ◉
Artificial tooth present   AT
Crown present   CR

Indicating the direction and
   extent of movement of teeth →
Bridge retainer present   BR
Bridge pontic present   BP
Primary teeth are indicated in the top right-hand corner of the appropriate
   square as ABCDE in diagrammatic charts without special provision for
   them.

Treatment records

A brief record of the treatment carried out must be made immediately after
the patient leaves the surgery while it is still fresh in the mind. This should
indicate the exact region, tooth or tooth surface involved, what was done,
and what materials or drugs were used. Any untoward occurrences during
treatment must be recorded in full detail.

Abbreviations. These are often used in practice, e.g. '6⌐ -MO ACR ID 2%
Xyl' means 'a Class II, mesio-occlusal cavity was prepared in the lower
right first permanent molar under inferior dental block anaesthesia
obtained with 2% xylocaine solution. The cavity was lined with cement and
restored with amalgam.'

The following list gives other examples of abbreviations commonly used
but they are not themselves standard and may vary from practice to
practice. The DSA must use and interpret them with great wariness to
avoid mistakes.

A	Amalgam
Ac	Acrylic
Ag	Silver
ANK	Appointment not kept
Au	Gold
C	Cement
DNA	Did not attend
F/- or FU	Full upper denture
-/F or FL	Full lower denture
GA	General anaesthetic
GDP	General dental practitioner
GMP	General medical practitioner
GP	Gutta percha
HSWMW	Hot salt water mouthwash
ID	Inferior dental block injection
Imps	Impressions
Inf	Infiltration injection
LA	Local anaesthetic

P/– or PU	Partial upper denture
–/P or PL	Partial lower denture
QS	Quick set
R	Restoration
RCT	Root canal therapy
SM	Study models
TCA	To come again
TP	Treatment plan
TTP	Tender to percussion
X	Extraction
ZnO	Zinc oxide (dressing)
#	Fracture (this sign also means 'Number', e.g. # 4)
⑥	Abscess (number denotes the tooth involved)

Other records

Various special diagnostic tests may be undertaken and the results must be carefully recorded and filed or stored as they become available.

Radiographs. Radiographs must always be labelled with the patient's name and the date upon which they were taken before they are filed. This also applies to photographic records.

Bulky records. Study models, specifically indicated working models, discarded dentures, etc, should be stored in labelled boxes to protect them from dust or breakage.

Laboratory tests. The results of laboratory investigation (biopsies, blood tests, bacteriological smears) should always be brought to the dental surgeon's immediate attention before they are filed away with the patient's records.

Chapter Seven

DENTAL RADIOGRAPHY

X-RAYS

X-rays are a radiation comparable to light and radio waves but differing from them in wavelength. They travel in a straight line from their source and can penetrate materials that are opaque to light, being deflected or absorbed by heavy atoms such as those found in metal and yet able to penetrate lighter atoms.

X-ray apparatus

X-rays are generated when a stream of electrons is stopped by impact with a solid. Inside a glass vacuum tube a heated wire filament (the cathode) generates a cloud of electrons which are accelerated by a high voltage electrical potential towards a shaped mass of metal (the anode) and focussed upon its surface. The energy of their impact generates x-rays which are emitted in all directions. Heat is also produced at the anode and so exposures are kept very short in duration and the vacuum tube is surrounded by a cooling jacket containing oil.

The tube is housed in a heavy metal screening cover which has a small window through which the working beam of x-rays is allowed to escape. The diameter of this beam can be limited and stopped down by a lead diaphragm and the central ray of the beam is arranged to pass through the point of a plastic centering cone on the x-ray machine's working head. The working head, which contains and covers the tube and its housing, is supported in a carefully counterbalanced positioning device that allows great flexibility of movement and angulation.

The apparatus has two warning lights: one to show that the machine is connected to the electrical mains and is 'live'; the second is a prominent and clearly visible indication of when x-rays are being generated. The x-ray set must be properly maintained to ensure that it does not continue to produce x-rays after the pre-set exposure has ended. The machine should always be switched off and 'dead' when not in use.

Dangers of exposure to x-rays

People working with x-rays are recommended to wear an exposure monitoring film badge to check that radiological safety standards are being maintained. Advice about such badges can be obtained from the local Department of Medical Physics.

Prolonged exposure to x-rays is very dangerous and the operator and others must make sure that they protect themselves by avoiding the direct beam and standing at least six feet away from the tube during exposures. No one other than the patient and the operator should remain in an x-ray room during the exposure unless this is essential, e.g. the mother to reassure a particular child. The x-ray beam should not be directed through thin walls into other areas or premises. Patients must not be exposed to x-rays beyond one full mouth examination (10 to 14 intra-oral films) a year, unless diagnostically necessary.

The x-ray beam should not be angled through the patient's trunk and must be directed away from the gonads. A pregnant woman patient should not be exposed at all to x-rays in the dental surgery if it can be avoided because of the danger to the developing cells of the unborn child. When an x-ray is essential in such a case, the mother and child must be protected with a special lead-rubber protective apron.

In no circumstances must the operator touch the cone or the tube housing, or hold a film in position in a patient's mouth during an exposure because the cumulative effects of such x-ray exposures can lead to radiation burns, skin ulceration, necrosis (death) of bone and loss of fingers.

In Great Britain the dental surgeon is accepted as a recognised radiation worker allowed to use x-rays in the dental surgery. The DSA may assist while radiographs are being taken, but is *not allowed* to use x-rays herself.

(*Note:* Exposure to the x-ray beam can 'de-programme' and spoil certain digital watches.)

Films

Ordinary photographic emulsion is sensitive to both light and x-rays. If a film, protected from light and moisture, is placed in the mouth on one side of the teeth and a beam of x-rays directed towards it from the other side, it passes through the teeth, bone and other tissues and throws a varying shadow on the film. The exposed film can then be developed in the dark room by ordinary photographic methods and will disclose details of the structures in and around the teeth that could not otherwise be examined.

Films may be *intra-oral* (e.g. peri-apical, occlusal, bite-wing) or *extra-oral* (e.g. lateral oblique).

Intra-oral films. The dental film packet for intra-oral use is supplied made up as follows:

1. A thin piece of tough transparent plastic film coated on both sides with a fine-grain photographic emulsion sandwiched between two thin sheets of black paper. (Some packets contain two pieces of film and the duplicate obtained is used for record purposes.)
2. This film is backed by a sheet of thin lead foil to prevent the x-rays from passing further and perhaps being reflected back from nearby structures and spoiling the film.
3. The outer envelope is made of light-proof paper and is labelled to indicate the side which should face away from the x-ray tube. This envelope is made up so that it can be opened easily in the dark room. (Some new films are contained in a simple plastic envelope only.)
4. In one corner of the film and repeated on the outer packet, there is a raised dot or pimple on the side that has to be towards the tube during exposure. This is of help in orientating the processed film correctly for viewing.

Extra-oral films. Large extra-oral films are usually exposed in light-proof, rigid metal cases called *cassettes*. When using extra-oral film, the x-rays have to pass through much denser areas of bone in the skull and, in order to increase their effect on the film without increasing the exposure time considerably, *intensifying screens* are fixed inside the cassette. These screens contain certain chemicals that glow and fluoresce when struck by x-rays right inside the light-proof cassette and this light further affects the film.

Extra-oral films must be orientated with a small lead letter 'L' or 'R' attached to the outside of the cassette before the exposure to indicate left or right. This letter will then be reproduced on the processed film.

All unexposed or undeveloped film must be protected from accidental x-ray radiation that will spoil it.

Making an exposure

1. The x-ray apparatus is switched on. Most machines are provided with a mains supply regulator so that the voltage may be adjusted to the recommended level before use.
2. The patient's head is positioned, resting it against a rigid support, e.g. the head rest of the dental chair.
3. The tube is placed in approximate position.
4. The film is placed in position.
5. The tube is adjusted to its accurate position.
6. The hand-timer, attached to the apparatus by a long cable, is set for the appropriate exposure time.

7. The operator and others retire to an appropriate distance behind the tube.
8. A visual check is made that nothing has moved and the patient warned to remain still.
9. The exposure release button is pressed firmly, noting that the exposure warning light on the apparatus comes on or, where provided, the milliammeter registers, while the exposure is made.
10. The intra-oral film is removed from the mouth and wiped dry as soon as possible to prevent saliva soaking through the paper envelope and affecting the film.

Exposure time will vary with the machine, the speed of the film that is used and the tissue penetration required. For example, with the average dental apparatus with an x-ray output at 10mA and 60kV, using a 9-inch focus-to-film distance and a fast film, intra-oral peri-apical films can be taken using exposures as short as 0.25 to 0.50 seconds.

Film positioning

Peri-apical films
1. The occlusal plane of the jaw to be radiographed should be horizontal.
2. The film packet is supported on the palatal or lingual side of the tooth with a special holder or forceps, so that the margin of the film just projects beyond the occlusal edge of the tooth and its sensitive side is towards the tube. The orientation pimple on the film packet should be kept towards the occlusal margin.
4. The tooth and the film are not parallel and to reduce distortion the central ray from the tube is directed at right angles to the plane, bisecting the angle between the axis of the tooth and the film (Fig. 7/1). The approximate vertical angle between the horizontal occlusal plane and the central ray for the various upper and lower teeth is shown in the chart below.

Peri-apical radiographs (Fig. 7/2)
Between 10 and 14 films are required to give full mouth peri-apical radiographs depending upon the system used to position the films.

Upper teeth	Vertical angle of x-ray tube	Lower teeth	Vertical angle of x-ray tube
$\underline{1}$	$+55°$	$\overline{1}$	$-20°$
$\underline{23}$	$+50°$	$\overline{23}$	$-20°$
$\underline{456}$	$+30°$	$\overline{456}$	$-10°$
$\underline{78}$	$+20°$	$\overline{78}$	$-\ 5°$

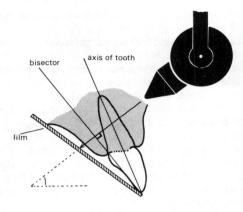

Fig. 7/1 Film and tube positioned for peri-apical radiography

Fig. 7/2 Peri-apical radiograph |5 6 7 8

Bite-wing films. A bite-wing film is obtained using a standard intra-oral film packet which has a paper flange or special holder attached to it along the occlusal plane. This holder is gripped between the teeth thus supporting the film firmly against the lingual and palatal surfaces of the upper and lower teeth at the same time. The tube is positioned with a 0° vertical angle from the occlusal plane. Only the crowns of the teeth will be shown on this film (Fig. 7/3).

Occlusal films. These are taken with larger intra-oral film packets held lightly between the occlusal surfaces of the upper and lower teeth with the sensitive side of the packet towards the tube.

The standard upper occlusal film. The central ray is directed from the bridge of the nose towards the mid-line of the palate at an angle of 60° to the occlusal plane.

The true upper occlusal film. The central ray is directed through the vertex of the skull towards the mid-line of the palate at 90° to the occlusal plane. A longer exposure time is required.

Fig. 7/3 Bite-wing radiograph (left side)

103

The lower occlusal film. The patient's head is extended and the tube is aimed upwards from below the chin at 90° to the occlusal plane.

Extra-oral films. These require larger films used in a cassette. The lateral oblique film is commonly taken to examine the molar region and ramus of the mandible. The cassette is supported against the angle of the mandible and cheek with the patient's head tilted as well as turned towards that side. The central ray can now be directed below the opposite angle of the mandible towards the molar region of the side under examination.

Other extra-oral films occasionally required include full lateral and postero-anterior skull films, films to show the maxillary antra and views of the temporomandibular joint.

Film processing (Fig. 7/4)

The exposed dental film or *radiograph* is processed in the same way as ordinary photographic film, usually in the dark room although daylight tanks or processors may be used in special circumstances.

Exposed films are *developed* with chemical solutions that carry on the work begun by the action of light or x-rays. The silver salts in the photographic emulsion that have been affected by the exposure are reduced to fine grains of metallic silver and then the film is *fixed* by further chemical action to remove the non-affected, unexposed silver salts in the other areas of the film.

Dark room procedures

The dark room excludes all normal daylight or artificial light that would affect the light-sensitive photographic emulsion. The only permissible light is from a special dim safelight fitted with an amber filter. Once one's eyes have become accustomed to this low glow the light is adequate for film processing procedures.

The standard solutions in the processing tanks must be well mixed and replaced regularly according to the manufacturer's instructions. The temperature of the solutions is important and should be checked with a thermometer and when necessary a special electric tank heater can be used.

When the dark room has been prepared the films are processed in the following way.

1. Lock the dark room door.
2. Switch off the ordinary light and put on the safelight.
3. Make sure that your hands are dry and clean.
4. Open the film containers one by one and clip the films in sequence on to the photographic hanger. Take care to hold the films by their edges only to avoid touching the emulsion. Up to 14 films may be placed on one hanger.

Fig. 7/4 Stages in processing intra-oral dental films

5. Label the hanger with the patient's name.
6. Put the discarded packet papers and lead foil into the appropriate waste receivers.
7. Put the films into the developer tank and agitate the hanger a little to prevent bubbles of air from remaining on the film surfaces and impeding the chemical action.
8. Put the light-proof lid on top of the developing tank.
9. Set the timing clock to indicate the developing time. This will be about four minutes at 20°C but depends upon the film speed, so check carefully.
10. When the developing time has elapsed lift the films from the developing tank and wash them in running water in the rinsing tank for 10 seconds to stop the chemical action.

11. Place the washed films into the fixing tank, again agitating them to remove air bubbles.
12. Reset the timing clock to indicate the fixing time. This varies from five to ten minutes, depending upon the chemical used.
13. When the films are fixed they are no longer light sensitive and the dim light can be exchanged for normal lighting.
14. After fixing the films are washed well in running water to remove all traces of chemicals and then hung up to dry in a dust-free atmosphere.

Note: Automatic film processing machines are now available to develop dental x-ray films. They require careful maintenance to ensure that the rollers are washed and clean and that the solutions are replaced regularly.

Faults

The following are some faults commonly met with and their most likely causes:

Film too dark: over-exposure or over-development
Film too light: under-exposure or under-development
No image: x-ray machine not switched on or fixing tank was inadvertently used first
Partial image: film in contact with another in tank
Fogged film: old film stock or light leak in dark room
Stained film: inadequate fixing or washing
Double image: patient or tube moved during exposure
Curved dark lines: film damaged by bending it

Orientating and mounting films

Intra-oral films are embossed in one corner with a raised pimple that is convex towards the tube (or the front of the film packet). By looking at the film as if from the outside of the patient's mouth, using the pimple as a guide, it is possible to orientate the film by the anatomy of the teeth depicted. Some dental surgeons store films in small envelopes while others prefer the films to be mounted on special sheets of transparent plastic or in cardboard mounts in their appropriate orientated positions for easy examination on the illuminated viewing box. Always write the patient's name on the envelope or mount immediately.

Chapter Eight

BASIC CONSERVATIVE DENTISTRY

Conservative dentistry is concerned with the operative techniques and materials used to restore carious, broken or worn natural teeth to normal function. More than half the time spent at the chairside in general practice is devoted to this type of treatment. This important and intricate work has to be carried out in the confined, dark, wet and sensitive environment of the mouth where each new restoration is immediately subjected to the destructive effects of masticatory pressures, moisture, temperature changes, various chemical activities and even the possibility of secondary carious attack. Instruments, materials and methods have been evolved to minimise or overcome these formidable difficulties.

THE OPERATING FIELD

The operating field has to be made as accessible and clearly visible as possible by positioning the patient's head properly, illuminating the mouth well, using a mouth mirror when necessary and by keeping the area dry. (Mouth mirrors may have plane or magnifying surfaces and may be attached to an electric mouth lamp to improve intra-oral illumination.)

A tooth can be kept dry by a variety of methods:

The saliva ejector with an appropriate tip attached. This will evacuate slowly saliva from the mouth, and works by water pressure.

The aspirator, both with a saliva ejector tip and a separate suction tip directed towards the tooth by the assistant. This will evacuate rapidly saliva, water and aerosol sprays from the mouth, and works by a vacuum generated by an electric pump.

Cotton wool rolls. These are placed in the buccal, labial or lingual sulcus to absorb saliva. These will work best when they are positioned near the appropriate salivary duct to absorb the saliva at its source.

Fig. 8/1 Rubber dam instruments

The rubber dam. A thin sheet of rubber is perforated with a rubber dam punch (Fig. 8/1) and applied to the appropriate teeth so that they protrude through the prepared holes. The sheet is retained on the teeth by special spring clamps or ligatured in place with waxed thread around the necks of the teeth. The edges of the dam are controlled by fastening them to a frame holder. The isolated teeth are thus kept free of moisture and contamination from the rest of the mouth during treatment and this method is commonly used during root canal therapy.

Air drying and wiping. The teeth may be dried by blowing air on them from an air syringe or by wiping them with a pledget of cotton-wool held in tweezers.

Anti-sialogogues. On rare occasions the mouth and teeth can be made drier if before the operation the patient is given a drug to reduce salivary flow.

HAND INSTRUMENTS
Dental probes (Fig. 8/2). These are sharp, pointed instruments that are made with a wide selection of curves and bends in their terminal shafts so that the tip may be more easily carried into remote places in the mouth.

PROBES

Briault

Fig. 8/2 Dental probes

They are used in conservative dentistry primarily to explore tooth surfaces, to locate cavities and wide pits and fissures and to search the prepared cavity surfaces to ensure that all traces of softened carious tooth substance have been eliminated.

Chisels (Fig. 8/3). These are used to split off unsupported enamel along the cleavage planes parallel to the enamel's prisms and also to plane down and smooth the cavity margins. Each type of chisel is made so that its cutting edge can be easily applied to the particular surface of the cavity for which it is intended. A *straight* chisel is exactly comparable with a wood-worker's chisel, although it is many times smaller, with the shaft in a straight line with the handle. *Angled* or *bin-angled* (having two bends or angles in the shaft) chisels are either *hoe* chisels (with their edge at right angles to the main shaft as in a garden hoe) or *hatchet* chisels (with their cutting edge in line with the main shaft like an axe). *Gingival margin trimmers* are hatchet chisels adapted for use in planing the cervical margins of interproximal cavities.

Excavators (Fig. 8/4). Softened, carious dentine can be removed from cavities by using hand excavators. These have small, spoon-shaped, circular (discoid) or oval (cleoid) tips which are very sharp around their circumference. They are pressed into the carious material and used to lever and dig out large fragments. When the bulk of the caries has been removed they can be used to scrape and explore the firmer surface of the prepared tooth to eliminate any final fragments. They allow good visibility during deep excavation of a tooth and are used when there is some danger of exposing the pulp.

109

Fig. 8/3 Dental chisels

Many different sizes of excavator tips are available and there are several basic angles of terminal shaft to allow them to be used more easily in different positions in the mouth.

THE DENTAL ENGINE

The quickest method of preparing cavities in teeth is by the use of rotating engine instruments powered by a dental engine that is usually controlled by a foot switch.

Fig. 8/4 Dental excavators

Electric engine. This is a variable-speed electric motor which drives the handpiece. Instrument speeds of from less than 500rpm up to 25 000rpm can be obtained and in some cases, specially geared engines connected to handpieces with high-speed bearings can be adjusted to develop 100 000rpm.

Air motor. This engine drive is directly adjacent to the handpiece and the motive power is produced by a slow air turbine fed by a simple tube conveying compressed air. This power system is very simple and the handpiece is relatively unrestricted in movement.

Air turbine. The motive power is again produced by compressed air passing through a turbine but now the turbine is a high-speed one and is actually in the head of the handpiece. Very high speeds of 250 000rpm to 300 000rpm can be obtained with this system and the handpiece bearings have to be lubricated constantly during use by a fine oil mist produced by dripping oil into the air-feed line.

HANDPIECES (Fig. 8/5)

These are of various types and are used to hold the engine-driven instrument firmly and transmit the motive power of the engine to it. They may be:

111

Fig. 8/5 Handpieces

Straight handpieces
Right-angled handpieces
Contra-angled handpieces
Miniature handpieces
Air turbine handpieces (always used with a water spray to prevent overheating of the tooth).

ENGINE INSTRUMENTS (Fig. 8/6)

These are made to be held in the various types of handpieces either by being gripped in a chuck or by a clip mechanism that fits into a special groove in the instrument's shank. Engine instruments are available in a range of materials and shapes to suit their various uses.

Materials
1. Steel.
2. Hardened tungsten carbide steel.
3. A steel shaft with a working head covered in diamond particles.
4. A steel shaft carrying a carborundum point or stone.

Fig. 8/6 Engine instruments

5. A steel mandrel to which may be attached a wide variety of discs or wheels (e.g. carborundum, diamond, rubber, sandpaper).
6. A steel shaft carrying a bristle brush or rubber tip.

Shapes
1. Burs (Fig. 8/7): Fissure (cross-cut fissure, tapered fissure), round (rose-head), inverted cone, wheel, end-cutting, finishing (which are smoother: round, pear, oval, flame shaped).
2. Diamond instruments: Bur shapes, fissure, round (rose-head), inverted cone, end-cutting both for conventional handpieces and air-rotors, wheels, discs, points.

113

Fig. 8/7 Burs

3. Stones: Green abrasive points, wheels and discs and white abrasive finishing points in many patterns.
4. Brushes and rubber polishing tips: Cup and wheel shapes.

CAVITY CLASSIFICATION

Cavities in teeth are generally classified according to the site of commencement of the carious process, as first proposed by Dr G. V. Black.

Black's classification
Class I – Cavities originating in anatomical pits, fissures and structural defects
Class II – Cavities originating on the proximal surfaces of molars and premolars
Class III – Cavities originating on the proximal surfaces of the incisors and canines and not involving the incisal angle
Class IV – Cavities originating on the proximal surfaces of incisors and canines and involving the incisal angle
Class V – Cavities originating on the gingival third of the labial, buccal, lingual or palatal surfaces of the teeth

CAVITY PREPARATION

All high-speed rotating engine instruments require that a water spray is used to cool the cut tooth surface during the operation. The DSA may be required to control the air and water sprays, and aspirate water and debris during the treatment, maintaining clear visibility of the tooth and protecting the patient's airway. This procedure generally follows the same sequence:
1. The *outline form* of the final cavity is planned and this depends upon the shape of the particular tooth.

2. The *convenience form* is considered as the tooth is opened up to allow easy access to the carious parts of the tooth that are to be removed.

3. The *resistance form* of the cavity is developed so that the final restoration will be able to withstand masticatory pressures, e.g. a flat floor to the cavity.

4. *Extension for prevention.* The cavity is extended to include any adjacent pits or fissures and thus prevent future caries attack at these weak points. Such extension is influenced by previous caries experience in the mouth and balanced by the need to conserve tooth substance.

5. The *retention form* is developed to ensure that the final restoration will be held firmly in the cavity.

6. All the remaining caries is removed from the cavity.

7. The margins of the cavity are smoothed and finished carefully.

Temporary restorations

After the cavity preparation has been completed it may not be convenient or even advisable to fill the tooth permanently at the same sitting in which case the tooth is dressed with a temporary filling. This must be non-irritant or even have a sedative effect, it should be quick-setting, firm when set, resistant to masticatory pressure and yet easily removed when necessary. Common temporary dressing materials include quick-setting zinc oxide cement, stiff zinc oxide and eugenol paste with or without incorporated cotton-wool filaments and, rarely, heat-softened gutta percha placed over an adequate lining layer of cement, for it is itself an irritant. Quick-setting zinc oxide cement contains zinc acetate which accelerates the setting time.

CAVITY LININGS

Before any permanent restoration is placed on top of a cut and prepared dentine surface a lining must be considered. Linings may be considered to have therapeutic and structural properties. Lining materials will protect the pulp from thermal or chemical influences during and after the introduction of the filling material and they can do much to support the tooth and restore the internal shape of the cavity. By covering the dentinal surface in this way internal staining of the tooth by amalgam is prevented.

Very deep cavities may be sub-lined with a calcium hydroxide cement to encourage the formation of secondary dentine in the pulp. Other lining cements are chosen because they are easy to manipulate, adhere to the walls of the cavity and set quickly enough for the final restoration to be packed upon them immediately without any possibility of the lining being displaced or crushed. Common lining cements include zinc phosphate cement and resin-reinforced quick-setting zinc oxide cement.

115

Very shallow cavities and certain cavity walls may be treated with cavity varnishes before an amalgam restoration is placed in position.

Mixing zinc phosphate cement

1. Portions of the cement powder and liquid are placed on a cold glass mixing slab. The liquid bottle must not be left open to the air for any longer than necessary or the water content will change and this will upset the properties of the cement and its setting times in future mixes.
2. The powder is divided into smaller portions with a metal mixing spatula.
3. Each small portion of cement powder is added to the liquid and thoroughly spatulated (mixed in) before the next portion is incorporated. The more slowly the first portions are added to the liquid, the longer the final setting time will be.
4. The whole mass is thoroughly mixed to incorporate as much powder as possible, to increase its strength and also to reduce its acid effect on the dentine and pulp.
5. The thick mix is transferred to the dried cavity and shaped with appropriate plastic instruments. To prevent the cement from sticking to the instruments they may be dipped in a small pile of dry cement powder or alcohol.

MATRICES

Where the cavity outline extends over more than a single surface of the tooth the final restoration material generally has to be packed into a box shape with one wall missing. In order to contain the filling material and allow it to be condensed properly a fourth wall has to be constructed temporarily as a matrix or shaper.

Types of matrix

Metal. A piece of thin stainless steel strip is held round the circumference of the tooth by a matrix holder or clamp. The band has to be held firmly against the tooth with wedges at the cervical margin in Class II cavities to prevent the filling material from extruding under packing pressure. Many different patterns of matrix holders are available.

Plastic. Thin plastic matrix strip is used to support most anterior filling materials, while they are being packed, held in place by the operator's fingers or with wedges and composition. Their transparency allows the operator to judge the position of the filling and any excess material at the cavity margins without having to disturb the matrix. Cellulose acetate or celluloid strips are used, but the latter reacts chemically with polymerising acrylic resin type materials.

Contoured matrices. Specially curved and shaped matrices can cope with particular problems such as the cervical margin or incisal edge restoration.

Plastic crown forms. Thin transparent crown forms are made in cellulose acetate and are used to control larger amounts of plastic restorative material, e.g. in the construction of temporary crowns, and for acid etch restorations of broken teeth.

'Compo' registers. Before the cavity is cut a piece of heat-softened composition is pressed over the tooth to record its shape and the margins of the adjacent teeth. This register, suitably protected with thin tinfoil or acetate sheet, can be used to form and support the final plastic filling material and thus ensure a true restoration of shape.

MIXING AND INSERTION OF THE FILLING MATERIAL

Plastic filling materials are soft and mouldable while they are being manipulated and packed into the prepared cavity in the tooth and then, within a short period of time, they harden and become resistant to displacement or fracture. Figure 8/8 illustrates some of the instruments used in filling prepared cavities.

Several different types of plastic filling materials are available. The commonest are silver amalgam and composite resins. The DSA should be familiar with the manufacturer's instructions for mixing the various filling materials which are in use in her particular practice.

Amalgam

Silver amalgam is an almost universal filling material that can be used in any class of cavity. It is not often used in the front of the mouth for aesthetic reasons. It is prepared by mixing together amalgam alloy (containing silver and tin with traces of copper and zinc), in a finely powdered form, with clean mercury in the following manner:

1. The proportions of alloy powder and mercury must be accurately dispensed by weight or other measuring system. Too much mercury causes the amalgam to expand excessively and reduces its flow and strength; too little mercury causes loss of working properties and porosity. A ratio of 1 part of alloy to 1.6 parts of mercury by weight is generally found to be the most suitable though the manufacturer's directions should be followed carefully.
2. The mix is prepared by combining the alloy powder and mercury in an

117

Stellite blade

SPATULAS

PLASTICS

amalgam
instruments

CARVERS

Frahm
90° R & L

Hampel improved

AMALGAM
CARRIERS

Ash

Fig. 8/8 Spatulas, plastics, carvers and amalgam carriers

automatic amalgam mixer when the soft amalgam presented will have a smooth, silvery appearance. Excessive mixing breaks down the crystal structure.

3. Small portions of the amalgam are conveyed to the dried cavity in an amalgam carrier and condensed into place with maximum pressure

using serrated amalgam pluggers or a mechanical engine condenser to bring excess mercury to the surface (Fig. 8/9).
4. Subsequent portions of amalgam are added to the first and condensed into place until the cavity is over-filled.
5. After the filling has hardened the excess material, which contains the surplus mercury, is cut away with carving instruments, any matrix is removed and the restoration is contoured to shape.
6. The restoration is checked for height of bite and general occlusion, adjusted as necessary by further carving and may then be smoothed with moist cotton-wool pellets.
7. Before he is dismissed the patient is warned to avoid heavy pressure or eating upon the restored tooth for at least an hour.

Health and safety note regarding the use of mercury

Mercury is poisonous. It can be *absorbed through the skin* and the hands should be washed immediately after handling anything that contaminates them with metallic mercury. At room temperature mercury vaporises into the air and can be *absorbed by inhalation*. Eating, drinking, smoking and the application of cosmetics should not be allowed in the dental surgery

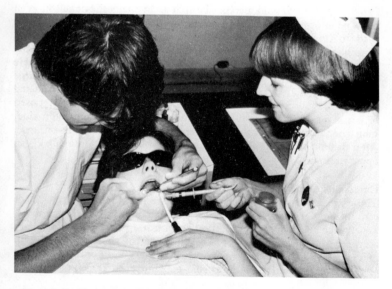

Fig. 8/9 Packing an amalgam restoration. The DSA is presenting the operator with further amalgam

because of the dangers of *absorption by swallowing* from mercury-contaminated hands and the environment. (Once the amalgam has set in the tooth all free mercury is fixed chemically and cannot poison the patient.)

The dental surgery should have efficient ventilation and working surfaces and floors should have hard, smooth surfaces with the minimum of crevices in which spilled mercury droplets could collect. Cleaning equipment and mops used on the surgery floor should not be used in other areas of the practice. A domestic vacuum cleaner must *never* be used in the dental surgery for this will rapidly raise the mercury vapour levels in the air.

All manipulations of mercury (e.g. mixing amalgam or transferring mercury from one container to another) should be carried out over a drip tray. All mercury, waste amalgam and other residues should be stored in well-sealed, non-metallic containers in a cool place. Waste should be covered with water in its collecting container to trap vapour. Waste must never be washed down the sink or left in a general waste bin. Waste mercury, amalgam and recovered spillage is valuable and when sufficient has accumulated it can be returned to the supplier for recovery.

Mercury spillage: Should mercury be spilt accidentally the dental surgeon must be informed immediately. Under his direction every effort must be made to recover every particle of the spilt mercury or to render it harmless. Equipment for dealing with spillage should be readily available in the practice and checked regularly. The kit usually consists of disposable plastic gloves, paper towels, a rubber bulb aspirator to draw up large globules of mercury, a container into which the mercury and contaminated items can be collected and sealed and a mercury absorbent paste (composed of equal parts of flowers of sulphur and hydrated calcium hydroxide, moistened with water) or a special proprietary substance for this purpose. After dealing with the spillage the room must be aired thoroughly via an open window.

Composite filling materials

These expensive materials consist of special resins which have up to 80 per cent of other materials added to them to improve their hardness, appearance and working properties. Such a resin differs from ordinary acrylic resin (it may be the reaction product of an epoxy resin with methacrylic acid). The additives may be tiny glass beads or rods, particles of quartz or lithium aluminium silicate. Unopened packets should be stored under refrigeration to extend shelf-life.

The shade and translucency of the basic material can be altered at the chairside when required by the addition of special colouring agents.

These materials are mainly used in Class III, IV and V restorations and, using the acid etch technique, in veneering and restoring stained, malformed or fractured teeth, periodontal splinting and orthodontic bonding.

For restorations:

1. The tooth is cleaned with an oil-free, non-fluoride polishing paste and rinsed thoroughly.
2. The cavity is prepared.
3. The tooth is isolated and dried.
4. The exposed dentine surfaces are lined and protected with an eugenol-free material such as a calcium hydroxide base.
5. The enamel walls of the cavity are etched with an acid solution, applied with a cotton-wool pledget, for 60 seconds. (Enamel on primary teeth requires two minutes' etching.)
6. The tooth is washed thoroughly with a water spray. (The patient must not rinse out or the etched surface will be contaminated with saliva.)
7. The tooth is isolated and dried thoroughly, when the etched surface will have a white frosty appearance.
8. The bonding layer components are mixed according to the manufacturer's instructions, usually on a paper pad with a plastic spatula provided in the kit, and applied to the etched surfaces.
9. The restorative filled resin is mixed and placed over the bond layer in the tooth, which does not have to have set first, and controlled as necessary by a matrix strip or crown form. Excess resin is best removed before setting occurs. Setting time, which is affected by room temperature, can be checked using the surplus mixture left on the paper mixing pad. *Note:* Some resins are 'light-cured' and only set when activated by intense light from a special source delivered by fibre-optic cable.
10. Any hard excess material is removed with rotating diamond instruments but the best results are obtained if such reduction can be kept to a minimum and the 'matrix shine' can be retained. (See also the acid etch technique of restoring borken teeth described on page 190.)

Note: Any acid accidentally contacting oral tissues, eyes or skin should immediately be flushed away with copious amounts of water. Uncovered etched enamel surfaces recover their normal appearance in a few days.

Retention pins

All plastic filling materials can be given better retention and reinforcement where necessary by the use of special metal pins. Basically, these are made of inert, threaded wire cut to an appropriate short length and, if necessary, bent into shape. The pins are cemented or threaded into prepared pinholes that have been drilled into the periphery of the cavity, away from the pulp, using special fine pinhole burs of the same diameter as the pin wire.

FINISHING AND POLISHING

Amalgam (after 48 hours)
(a). The bite height is checked with articulating paper when necessary.
(b). The surface is smoothed with engine-driven stones, finishing burs and sandpaper discs.
(c). The interproximal surfaces are polished with linen polishing strips by hand.
(d). The whole surface is polished with pumice powder and water paste on engine-driven rubber cups and bristle brushes.
(e). The final polish is completed with a whiting and alcohol paste applied with a clean, soft brush, rotating at high speed and light pressure.

Composite filling materials (after the recommended time)
(a). The bite is checked.
(b). Any bulk excess is removed with rotating diamond stones.
(c). The surface may be smoothed, if necessary, with white mounted stone points, followed by various grades of flexible Soflex polishing discs.

Chapter Nine

INLAYS, CROWNS AND BRIDGEWORK

In addition to the plastic restoration techniques in which the materials are packed, moulded, allowed to harden and finished in the prepared tooth, other restorations can be fabricated outside the mouth on models and then cemented into place. Care and precision and the highest standards of work are necessary if this complex type of treatment is to meet with success.

INLAYS

An inlay is a cast gold restoration shaped to fit accurately into a cavity prepared in the crown of a tooth. They are used most commonly to restore badly broken down posterior teeth that have to withstand considerable masticatory pressure or to support bridges.

In general an inlay cavity when prepared and lined must have retentive almost parallel walls without any undercuts, sharp internal cavity angles and should have a flat seating floor. Where appropriate the enamel margins at the cavo-surface angle around the periphery of the cavity are bevelled, e.g. at the occlusal and gingival margins. This will remove weakened enamel prisms and also improve the marginal fit of the final restoration, because gold has a good edge strength and 'feather-edge' produced can be burnished in this region. The main retention of the finished inlay comes from its overall sliding fit into the cavity assisted by the grip and locking effect of the final cementing medium. The line of withdrawal should, when possible, be in the line of, and in the opposite direction to the stresses likely to be placed upon it in the mouth. Still further retention can be obtained when necessary by the use of pins and ridges cast onto the basic inlay that will fit into prepared pinholes (see Fig. 9/2) and slots cut into the tooth.

Basically, inlay preparations can be described using Black's Classification although it is unusual to construct Class I inlays in occlusal surfaces. Modern dentistry finds little indication for simple inlays (Fig. 9/1), and the method now tends to be reserved for cases where the cusps of the

Fig. 9/1 Class I gold inlay cavity
on a premolar

Fig. 9/2 Class II inlay preparation in a
premolar. Note the retention pin

tooth are undermined, weakened or lost and full cuspal coverage or
replacement with gold is required. In situations where a minimal amount of
tooth needs to be removed interproximally a 'slice-preparation' is used
(Fig. 9/2).

IMPRESSION TECHNIQUES

Direct impressions

A piece of inlay wax is heated in a flame, pressed into the prepared cavity,
cooled and then trimmed and contoured to the correct shape and occlusion.
In complex cavities the inlay wax may have to be controlled in the first
instance with a metal matrix band positioned around the tooth. Once the
pattern has been satisfactorily prepared it may be removed from the cavity
with a probe or sprue, taking care not to bend or distort the wax. The wire
sprue is heated and attached to the pattern at its thickest point, well away
from its edges or fitting surface, before sending it to the laboratory for
immediate investment and casting (see Laboratory Technique, p. 126).
This technique requires special skill, can really only be used for very simple
inlays which then require time-consuming polishing in the mouth, and is
mainly superseded by the indirect methods.

Indirect impressions

This is the best method for making complex multi-surface inlays
particularly in inaccessible regions of the mouth. An accurate impression of
the cavity and adjacent teeth is taken, together with a record of the shape of

the opposing teeth and registration of occlusion. Models are then prepared in the laboratory, mounted in articulation, and the inlay is constructed on them. This method demands special care in the impression and model making stages to ensure that small inaccuracies cannot occur that will spoil the fit of the finished inlay.

Copper ring and composition. A short length of soft copper tube (called a ring or band) of the correct size to fit round the circumference of the tooth is selected. The ring is cut to shape with crown scissors and green abrasive stones and contoured with pliers until it fits the tooth snugly and extends just beyond the margins of the cavity and avoids undercut regions. This will ensure that the composition it will later contain cannot get trapped in such undercuts and, setting hard, cause difficulty and distortion when the impression is removed. The ring is filled with inlay impression composition that has been heated to working softness in a flame. The ring and composition is placed accurately on the tooth and pressed home firmly. The composition is cooled with a stream of cold water and the impression is removed carefully, without rocking, to avoid distortion. An impression of the adjacent and opposing teeth is taken, often simply in softened pink wax that has aluminium-filled wax added to the side in contact with the preparation to give greater detail in that region.
Note: Other impression materials besides composition can be used in a copper ring.

Elastic impressions. Various non-reversible elastic impression materials are available that are based on mercaptan or silicone rubbers. These materials are creamy when mixed, but set into a tough, stable, rubbery and elastic consistency that will give extremely accurate detailed impressions of inlay and crown preparations and the adjacent teeth and tissues. They can reproduce undercuts. Using these materials and a careful technique, several inlay cavities may be prepared in the same quadrant of the mouth at once and with a single impression all the inlays completed and fitted at the second appointment.

These materials are usually presented as two pastes, one containing the accelerator or catalyst, or as a paste and a liquid that has to be dispensed from a dropper. The working consistencies can be varied from thick to thin. A special tray should be constructed for each case and this must be coated with the tray adhesive to hold the material in place. The cavity is isolated and the gingival tissues retracted away from the margins with an astringent packing string which is removed before the impression is taken. This is necessary to prevent gingival oozing and also because the paste flows into place without pressure and would be easily deflected by the untreated gingival tissue overhanging cavity margins. The cavity is dried carefully.

125

The measured amounts of impression material and activator are mixed thoroughly, usually with a spatula on a disposable paper pad. In complex cavities, thin impression material may be conveyed to the deeper, inaccessible places by a syringe or a plastic instrument to eliminate the possibility of trapped air, but the bulk of the thicker impression material is carried into place in the tray. The setting time is observed accurately before the impression is removed and checked. An impression is taken of the opposing teeth, usually in alginate. Best results are obtained when full mouth impressions are taken and the models articulated into a wax leaf bite registration to avoid inaccuracies of occlusion.

Temporary restorations
These are very important to protect the tooth, stabilise its position and prevent gingival overgrowth during the period of inlay construction. The material used must be easily and cleanly removable at the next appointment.

LABORATORY TECHNIQUE

Briefly, the impression must be cast into accurate, hard, working models. The prepared tooth model may be cast individually in extra-hard stone or produced by copper plating. The resultant tooth model or die is then seated into the larger impression of the arch and the whole model can then be cast up and articulated with the model of the opposing teeth. Some operators prefer that the model should be cast in one stage to avoid seating errors of such pre-cast dies.

The inlay pattern is waxed up on the die, sprued with a length of wire and removed from the model. At this stage, both the direct wax and the indirect proceed in the same way (Fig. 9/3).

The wax pattern to be cast is coated with a layer of semi-liquid investment material which is similar in consistency to dental plaster. The coated pattern is then set in a metal casting ring and surrounded by further investment material. Great care must be taken to avoid air bubbles in the investment that would spoil the final casting, and these are eliminated by vibration or vacuum techniques.

When the investment has set, the sprue is removed and the ring and its contents heated in a furnace. The wax melts and burns away leaving a space into which molten gold can be cast.

The casting is then cleaned, polished, fitted to the model and returned to the surgery.

Fig. 9/3 The laboratory stages of making an inlay by direct and indirect methods

127

FITTING AND CEMENTING THE INLAY

The temporary dressing is removed from the cavity and the inlay tried in to check the fit, the margins, the bite height and the contact points with the adjacent teeth. Any minor adjustments can be made at the chairside and the gold repolished, but with an accurate technique and careful work in the laboratory this should rarely be necessary. The gold margins are burnished carefully to ensure that they are perfectly adapted to the tooth surface. The inlay is washed in alcohol to remove any grease from polishing or handling it and dried. The cavity is washed and the tooth isolated with cotton-wool rolls and saliva ejector and dried with a jet of warm air. A thin mix of zinc phosphate cement is prepared and some is coated over the fitting surface of the inlay before more is carried to the tooth surface with an instrument. Thus the higher temperature of the tooth, which accelerates the cement setting time, will not be a problem. The inlay is placed in position in the mouth and pressed well home with an instrument. Some dental surgeons like to tap the inlay home with an automatic mallet. If necessary the inlay may be held in place by getting the patient to bite on a wood point (the kind used for interdental cleansing) positioned over the inlay. When the cement has set, the extruded excess is removed from all the margins and between the teeth with a probe and floss silk. The result should be an inlay with its margins in firm accurate contact with the tooth and no cement line.

CROWNS

A crown is a very extensive restoration of the coronal structure of a tooth. They may be prepared on anterior or posterior teeth and are classified according to their design or the material of which they are made.

Jacket crowns

These are generally used on anterior teeth for they can give a very good aesthetic appearance.

Porcelain (Fig. 9/4). The whole enamel surface of the tooth is removed with diamond instruments to leave a dentine peg protecting the pulp, and a cervical shoulder is prepared. A full arch impression in rubber is taken as for an inlay together with an alginate impression of the opposing teeth and an accurate colour shade record. In the laboratory the porcelain crown is constructed by fusing together tinted porcelain powders on a die-prepared platinum matrix in a special furnace and finally glazing the surface. The platinum lining the finished crown must be removed before it is cemented into place. Very accurate and detailed colour matches can be obtained and the slightly translucent porcelain looks exactly like natural enamel.

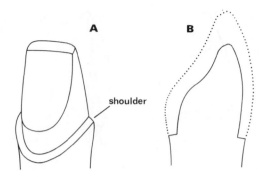

Fig. 9/4 A. Incisor prepared for a porcelain jacket crown
B. Lateral aspect to show outline of the finished crown

Porcelain bonded to gold. In this method the preparation needs a wider labial shoulder than for a porcelain jacket crown, but does not require a wide cervical shoulder on the palatal or interproximal surface because these regions of the crown are covered with a veneer of gold. Porcelain is heat bonded to the labial and incisal surfaces of the gold to give a good aesthetic result. (Acrylic may also be used in this way but is less resistant to wear and not as colour-fast.)

Post crowns

When all the coronal structure of the tooth is lost, or the tooth weakened by root canal therapy or very extensive caries, any crown has to be made on a central reinforcing post or post and core.

Post or dowel crown. The natural crown is removed to gingival level and the root canal cleaned of filling to an adequate depth to hold the post. The surface of the remaining tooth substance is prepared to support the crown and prevent it from rotating. In one of several possible techniques an impression of both the prepared root face and the root canal may be taken together. The usual locating impressions, bite and tooth shade are required.

Post and core. In this method the post is made first and cemented into place before the crown is constructed (Fig. 9/5). After preparing the canal as before, a wire of wrought gold or other suitable metal is waxed up as necessary to fit the canal and to produce a coronal extension similar in shape to the final crown preparation. Additional gold is cast on to the wire in the

129

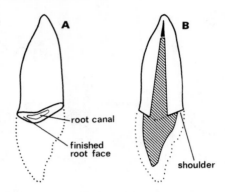

Fig. 9/5 A. Incisor ready for gold post and core
B. Gold post and core fitted and prepared for a porcelain jacket crown. The tooth
has been apically sealed with a sectioned silver point

laboratory and the post and core cemented into place. A conventional full
crown preparation is made and a jacket crown constructed and cemented
into place.

Three-quarter crowns

These are really extensive veneer gold inlays used to reinforce weakened
teeth or to make a firm abutment for a bridge. Three-quarters of the surface
of the tooth may be removed in this preparation (Fig. 9/6), together with
the incisal edge or the occlusal surface, but commonly leaving the buccal or
labial enamel untouched for appearance. Retention is gained with
interproximal slots or pins placed so that the final crown is inserted from
the incisal or occlusal direction. Ideally, retention grooves should be placed
as far buccally as possible to achieve the greatest length and effect. (The
chamfer or bevelled shoulder is becoming less popular because its feather
edge may lead to wax distortion and casting defects in this region.)

Fig. 9/6 Three-quarter crown preparation on a molar from the mesial aspect

Fig. 9/7 A. Full veneer crown preparation on a molar from the mesial aspect
B. Section from the buccal aspect with tooth in situ and crown fitted

Full crowns

Badly broken down posterior teeth can be restored with full gold crowns covering all clinical surfaces (Fig. 9/7). The preparations can be shoulderless or to a shoulder. Full crowns of this kind can be constructed on pinned amalgam cores for badly destroyed teeth and will do much to support weakened enamel and dentine by giving *extra-coronal retention* around the outside of the tooth. The impression technique is broadly that described for indirect inlays.

Temporary crown restorations

These are very important for aesthetic reasons, to protect and stabilise the tooth and also to hold back the gingival margins.

Temporary crowns may be constructed of acrylic in the laboratory to impressions taken before the preparations are made, they may be made with pre-formed crown forms filled with acrylic or other plastic (e.g. Scutan) at the chairside, or from cold-cure acrylic materials shaped between the prepared tooth and a pre-preparation alginate impression. The crowns are fixed with temporary cement. Posterior teeth can also be protected with selected and marginally trimmed aluminium crown forms filled with quick-setting zinc oxide cement.

Fitting and cementing the crown

The technique is similar to that used for an inlay. The margins, occlusion, overall contour, contact points, shade and general appearance are checked, and for anterior crowns the patient should also be allowed to examine and

131

approve the appearance before the crown is finally cemented into place with zinc phosphate cement.

BRIDGES

Dental bridges are non-removable appliances constructed to restore a missing tooth or teeth and attached to the adjacent sound teeth. The foundation teeth are prepared for inlays or crowns, *abutments*, to support the span of the bridge, the *pontic*.

Bridge pontics may be rigidly fixed to the abutment at each end, *fixed-fixed*, or they may have an interlocking attachment at one end that allows a little independent movement between the abutment teeth, *fixed-movable* (Fig. 9/8.) Prefabricated precision attachments are available to help in planning and constructing the movable attachment.

Fig. 9/8 A fixed-movable bridge with sanitary pontic filling saddle area in the position of the first molar

Assessment and design

Before a bridge can be constructed the mouth has to be assessed clinically, as well as by study models and radiographs to check and consider such things as the periodontal health, the strength of the root attachments, the caries rate, the occlusion, the span of the proposed bridge, and so on, before a design can be made. Not every case is suitable.

TYPES OF BRIDGE

Anterior bridges. These are usually constructed for aesthetic purposes to replace a lost tooth. All gold in the abutment teeth is kept as invisible as possible using tooth-coloured facings where necessary. The abutments may be inlays usually with full cuspal coverage, three-quarter crowns or full crowns depending upon the shape, position and condition of the supporting teeth. *Cantilever* bridges may be indicated in which a crown on a posterior tooth, e.g. premolar or canine, supports an anterior tooth, e.g. a central incisor, on a firm gold bar curving forward and out of sight behind the teeth. This puts considerable strain and leverage on the posterior tooth. *Spring cantilever* bridges have a similar design but a more flexible gold bar is used that gains some support from the underlying mucosae (Fig. 9/9).

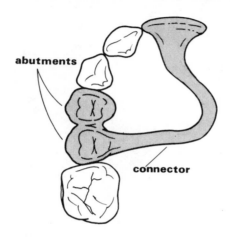

Fig. 9/9 Spring cantilever bridge designed to replace missing central incisor. Full gold crowns on the premolars with a soldered joint between them act as the abutment

Posterior bridges. Here the main requirement is to provide a good masticatory surface for the opposing teeth to work against. Sturdy abutment teeth are essential and often full gold crowns are used. Where the aesthetic appearance is not important a *sanitary pontic* is used in which a space is left between the occlusal working surface and the mucosa to allow the tongue and normal oral hygiene methods better access for cleaning under the bridge (Fig. 9/8).

Technique of bridge construction
1. Assess the case and plan the bridge.
2. Prepare the abutment teeth.
3. Take impressions of the abutment teeth.
4. Take the bite, shade and impression of the opposing teeth.
5. Place the temporary restorations.

133

6. Try in the abutment restorations.
7. Take a locating impression of the abutments.
8. Place further temporary restorations.
9. Try in the completed bridge.
10. Cement the bridge into place.
11. Show the patient how to clean the bridge properly.
12. Follow-up at intervals to check function.

Chapter Ten

PULP TREATMENT AND ROOT CANAL THERAPY

The restoration of teeth is often complicated by the proximity of the advancing carious process to the pulp. When the caries extends into the pulp chamber, acute or chronic inflammation, *pulpitis*, abscess or death of the pulp, *pulpal necrosis*, will occur and the infective process may proceed further to cause peri-apical infection. Sometimes, if the patient does not receive treatment, the pain and discomfort of this infective process can settle down to a painless chronic condition that no longer seems to him to require attention. Untreated dead teeth or chronic apical infection have long been regarded as a continual hazard to the patient's general health, particularly in cases with heart valve lesions, etc. By modern pulp treatment, root canal therapy (*endodontics*) and apical surgery techniques, infection and chronic apical inflammation can be eliminated in many cases, otherwise the affected tooth will have to be extracted.

Case selection

A non-vital tooth may be selected for pulp or root canal therapy in a co-operative patient who has no medical contra-indications, whose general oral condition merits this treatment, where the tooth is of value for appearance, masticatory or denture or bridge support reasons and where the individual tooth's condition gives a good chance of success.

Pulp diagnosis

1. Case history of any pain, noting its onset, intensity and duration.
2. Clinical examination noting any cavity, fracture, local apical swelling, inflammation or sinus, tenderness to percussion or looseness in the socket.
3. Special tests:
   (a) Pulp vitality tests with heat (hot gutta percha) and cold (ice or evaporating ethyl chloride on cotton-wool) or with the electric pulp tester.

(b) Radiographic examination to observe the depth of the cavity, the anatomy of the root canal and the peri-apical condition.

(c) Excavation of the cavity to see if there is an opening into the pulp chamber (pulp exposure).

TREATMENT METHODS

Pulpitis

Painful inflammation of the unexposed pulp can sometimes be resolved in its earliest stages by removing the cause (exposed dentine, caries, chemical or thermal irritants) and filling the cavity with a sedative dressing, such as zinc oxide and eugenol paste, for a few days.

Pulp capping

This is carried out on a vital tooth where a small, non-infected exposure of the pulp has occurred. The exposure is covered with a calcium hydroxide and sterile water paste that will encourage the formation of secondary dentine to seal the breach and maintain the vitality of the pulp. The tooth is filled permanently and tested at intervals in later months to ensure that the pulp remains healthy.

Pulpotomy

When the exposure is large and potentially infected the crown pulp is removed under anaesthesia and sterile conditions leaving vital, non-infected pulp tissue undisturbed in the root canal. In young patients this may allow an unformed tooth apex to continue to grow normally. The amputated surface is covered with calcium hydroxide paste and the tooth filled permanently. It should be kept under regular radiographic survey in case the tooth requires conventional root treatment subsequently.

Pulpectomy

When the whole pulp is infected it becomes necessary to remove the total contents of the pulp chamber both in the crown and root or roots. The tooth is anaesthetised if necessary and then isolated with rubber dam and a good saliva ejector. The surface of the tooth is sterilised with a disinfectant solution and the tooth is opened with sterile burs. Once access to the root canal is gained the pulp is removed with a fine barbed broach passed up into the canal and rotated to catch and hold the pulp tissue.

Drainage

When pulpal inflammation has proceeded to pus formation some peri-apical swelling and infection may occur. In these circumstances it may be necessary to leave the tooth open to drain away the pus and inflammatory exudates for 24 hours or so before the root canal therapy can be continued. With severe infections general supportive treatment and antibiotics may be indicated.

Measurement of root canal length

An accurate determination of the length of a root canal can be made by taking a radiograph of it while a metal root canal instrument of known length lies inside the tooth. By measuring the apparent length of the known instrument and the apparent length of the unknown root canal on the radiograph, the working length of the root canal can be calculated by simple proportion.

Preparation of the root canal

The canal has to be cleaned to eliminate infected dentine, enlarged, all debris removed and the canal rendered sterile before a permanent root filling can be put into it.

Instrumentation. The walls of the root canal are cleaned and prepared using reamers and files (Fig. 10/1). *Reamers* are worked by a rotary action either by hand or in a handpiece with the dental engine running at slow speed.

Smooth   Barbed   Engine   FILE   ROTARY PASTE FILLER

BROACHES   REAMERS

Fig. 10/1 Broaches, reamers, files and rotary paste fillers

137

Their spiral cutting action tends to work debris downwards towards the coronal end of the root canal. *Root canal files* have serrated surfaces and are inserted into the root canal, pressed against one wall at a time and scraped out again to remove debris. Sets of reamers and files are graded in diameter sizes and are used in an ascending sequence to gradually enlarge and prepare the root canal. These instruments are also made in various lengths to cope with teeth of different sizes. Not every root canal can be penetrated completely for there may be mechanical problems due to curvatures or calcified blockages. Ideally the canal is reamed to a length 0.5mm short of the apex, a point of natural constriction in most mature teeth.

Asepsis. All root canals must be clean, dry and sterile before they are filled; infection must be eliminated for the patient's safety. Treatment is carried out using an aseptic technique with rubber dam in place to avoid contamination from the mouth. All instruments and materials used in the root canal must be sterile. Root canal therapy boxes may be made up containing all the instruments, cotton-wool, paper points, etc, sterilised and kept immediately available for treatment. Infected debris is washed away from the canal with narrow-bore needles on a sterile syringe using sterile saline solution or dilute hydrogen peroxide solution followed by a solution of sodium hypochlorite. Fluid may be removed from the root canal with dry paper points which are absorbent. Disinfection of the canal is achieved by placing a paper point or cotton-wool pledget in the tooth moistened with a disinfectant such as camphorated parachlorophenol and sealing it firmly into place for several days. Such a root canal dressing may have to be repeated at intervals until the canal is sterile. Bacteriological tests for sterility may be carried out by placing a sterile paper point in the canal for one minute to absorb any exudate and then dropping it into a broth culture medium to see if any organisms have survived and can be cultured during the next day or so in an incubator.

Filling the root canal
Once the canal has been prepared and sterilised it may be filled permanently (*obturated*) with a solid point of correct diameter and length, usually made of gutta percha or silver, sealed into place with a suitable cement. The walls of the canal are dried and then the canal is filled with a thin, creamy mix of slow-setting cement carried into place either by hand, using a reamer in reverse rotation, or with an engine-driven rotary paste filler (Fig. 10/1). The core point is then carried up into place to its predetermined length. Additional accessory gutta percha points may be needed to pack laterally against the main point once it is in position. Finally, all the excess lengths of points still projecting from the cavity are cut off level with the opening of the canal and the cavity filled before

removing the rubber dam. A check radiograph is taken immediately to confirm that the root filling is adequate, and the canal is filled to the apical constriction with no visible voids along its length.

Follow-up

All root-treated teeth are kept under routine clinical and radiographic observation to make sure that apical infection does not recur. Radiographs are taken at three months, six months and then annually for about five years to ensure that all is well.

Apical surgery

When apical infection cannot be permanently eradicated by root canal therapy, apical surgery will be necessary if the tooth is to be safely retained in the mouth. The infected apex is either scraped (*curetted*) or cut off and removed (*apicectomy*) and the apical granulation curetted away (see Oral Surgery, p.167).

Chapter Eleven

PERIODONTOLOGY

Periodontology is the branch of dentistry concerned with the prevention and treatment of diseases involving the periodontal tissues. Periodontal disease (pyorrhoea), like dental caries, has an almost universal distribution throughout the human race and its incidence increases steadily with age. The real danger lies in the fact that it can cause slow, insidious and often painless deterioration of the supporting structures of the teeth which all too often remains unrecognised until treatment can no longer be effective and teeth are lost. Age-related surveys have shown that while dental caries is responsible for most of the extractions carried out in the first two decades of life, in later years the periodontal diseases become increasingly important. In the age-group 35 to 40 years they are responsible for more than 60 per cent of all extractions and this figure rises to over 80 per cent in people of 65 years and older. Early diagnosis is essential if treatment is to be effective and it must be borne in mind that the first stages of disease can often be detected in adolescence.

PERIODONTAL DISEASE

This is the general term used to describe plaque-induced disease of the periodontium or supporting structures of the teeth (the cementum, the periodontal membrane, the alveolar bone and the overlying gingival tissues).

Gingivitis

This is inflammation of the gingival tissues and is usually the first stage in the onset of periodontal disease. It may arise from a variety of local and general causes.

Local causes. The common local causes are all conditions that lead to poor oral hygiene and subsequent plaque accumulation leading to a constant irritation of the gingivae:

1. Inefficient tooth brushing and food stagnation.
2. A consistently soft diet that does nothing to stimulate and harden the gingival tissues.
3. Heavy tobacco smoking which tends to be associated with poor oral hygiene.
4. Irregularly arranged teeth, traumatic bites or unopposed teeth.
5. Untreated dental caries or inadequate or badly contoured restorations.
6. Ill-fitting dentures or orthodontic appliances.
7. Drying due to mouth-breathing.

Gingivitis is thus associated with the presence of plaque and calculus on the teeth and in the gingival crevice.

Plaque. Where oral hygiene is poor, dental plaque can build up rapidly in the gingival crevice. The plaque contains certain components which cause dental caries, and others which initiate periodontal disease. The products of this plaque are very irritant to the gingivae, causing inflammation and degeneration of the deeper tissues with irreversible breakdown and pocket formation. The deeper layers of established plaque can mineralise to form calculus.

Plaque index. There are several methods of scoring the extent of plaque present on the teeth. One is based on calculating a simple percentage of the number of tooth surfaces with plaque present, against the number of tooth surfaces available. Each tooth is scored as having four surfaces thus excluding the occlusal.

Calculus (tartar). This is commonly found in association with gingivitis and periodontal disease. It is a soft, yellow-white, porous material which hardens and stains with time. It can occur on teeth anywhere in the mouth but forms particularly on tooth surfaces that lie close to the openings of the salivary ducts: on the buccal sides of the maxillary molars opposite the parotid ducts and on the lingual surface of the mandibular incisors opposite the sublingual ducts. Calculus is made up of about 70 per cent inorganic material and 30 per cent organic matter and water by weight. It is composed mainly of calcium phosphate and carbonate with traces of magnesium and other elements together with bacteria, epithelial cells and debris.

Supragingival calculus forms on the parts of the teeth that are visible above the gingival margin and *subgingival calculus* forms just below the gingival margin.

When plaque and calculus are removed from the teeth the local gingival inflammation resolves in most cases.

General factors. There may also be general factors involved that predispose to gingivitis such as vitamin deficiencies, blood disorders, hormonal changes, e.g. in pregnancy, and the use of certain drugs. It has also been reported that certain races are more susceptible to gingival diseases than others.

Acute inflammation of the gingival and periodontal tissues may be caused by local infections which are painful and require urgent treatment, e.g. *acute ulcerative gingivitis* and *pericoronitis* which are discussed later, but generally gingival inflammation passes unnoticed into the chronic stage.

At first, in *chronic gingivitis*, the gingival margins are very slightly swollen and may bleed easily. If the disease is neglected the inflammation gradually spreads deeper to involve the periodontal membrane, etc. The condition may now be clinically termed chronic marginal periodontitis; the swollen gingivae become detached from the necks of the teeth and a true pocket is formed in which further food debris, plaque, calculus and inflammatory products can accumulate. This serious condition is usually painless and may also pass unnoticed by the patient although his near acquaintances will be aware that he has bad breath, *halitosis*.

Gradually, if still untreated, the gingival attachment recedes towards the apical region of the tooth, the pockets enlarge, the fibres of the periodontal membrane are progressively destroyed, the gingivae recede, and, at the same time, the alveolar bone of the socket is resorbed until finally the tooth loosens (see Fig. 3/3, p.67).

Diagnosis

A detailed case history is taken with particular attention to the patient's gingival symptoms (bleeding gums, loosening teeth, etc), general health and medical and drug history. Special information is sought about the oral hygiene, dietary and smoking habits which all have a direct effect on the gingival and periodontal health.

The oral examination first records the general overall condition of the mouth, noting the oral hygiene, standard of conservation treatment and occlusion before proceeding to the detailed examination of the oral mucosa and teeth. A detailed record is made of the condition of the gingivae, the presence of calculus, the presence and extent of pocketing around the teeth, the mobility and occlusion of the individual teeth. The presence of dentures, bridgework or other appliances is noted. A specialised chart can be used to record the condition of the patient's periodontal structure by indicating the depth of pockets on a 2mm horizontal line or grid system (see Fig. 6/2, p.93). The pocket depth can be measured accurately with a calibrated periodontal probe.

A radiographic examination to assess the alveolar bone loss follows and models or bacteriological and blood tests may be required to complete the diagnosis.

TREATMENT

Initial preparation

This is aimed at eliminating as many of the causative factors as possible. It is essential that the patient deals with such matters as poor oral hygiene and attention to diet and general health. Acute conditions may require the use of antibiotics as well as local cleansing or even extraction to eliminate pain and infection. Once the condition of the mouth begins to improve, the results of previous neglect and damage can be tackled in the dental surgery.

Scaling and polishing

All plaque and calculus must be removed from the teeth if their irritant effects are to be overcome. Calculus, both supra- and sub-gingival, is cleaned from the teeth by scaling. Scaling instruments are designed to be used to search out and remove calculus and to plane the tooth sub-gingivally to render its surface smooth. A very wide range of shapes of scalers is obtainable, but most dental surgeons confine themselves to a small number, perhaps half a dozen, that they personally find adequate for the purpose.

Scaling instruments (Fig. 11/1) fall into four main categories:

1. *Chisel or push scalers.* These have a thin flexible end, tipped with a sharp blade, and are used to pass between the anterior teeth and dislodge calculus attached to their proximal surfaces.

2. *Sickle scalers.* These have blades that are triangular in cross-section and are used to remove supra-gingival calculus. The edge of the blade is carried below the gingival margin and the calculus is dislodged by pulling the instrument coronally while holding the blade firmly against the surface of the tooth.

3. *Hoe scalers.* These are used mainly for the removal of sub-gingival calculus. The short blade projects at right angles to the shaft of the instrument. The tip of the hoe is inserted into the pocket with the sharp surface towards the tooth, the calculus located by touch, the blade engaged and the material removed by a pull stroke.

4. *Curettes.* These are planing instruments, similar in shape to oval (cleoid) dentine excavators, used for removal of deep deposits of calculus and contaminated cementum.

All scaling instruments must be kept sharp, and to assist this some of the hoe scalers are made with extra-hard tungsten carbide tips.

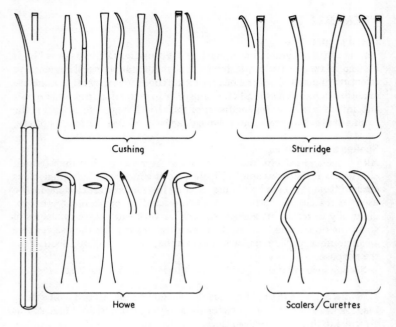

Fig. 11/1 Scaling instruments

Ultrasonic scalers. The apparatus can be separate or built into the dental unit, and has a lead to a special scaling handpiece. A sterilised insert with a scaler tip, is placed into the handpiece and can be made to vibrate ultrasonically at 25 000 vibrations per second. The instrument will effectively remove calculus deposits from the teeth by both mechanical and ultrasonic activity. Several types of insert are available, each with a different action. Ultrasonic scaling is always carried out under a water spray for cooling and lavage. This requires efficient aspiration using high-speed suction.

Root planing. In cases where there is established pocket formation, full mouth root planing will be required under local anaesthesia. The aim is to remove hard deposits and contaminated cementum from sub-gingival root surfaces.

After the scaling has been completed, polishing can be carried out to remove remaining stains and to smooth the tooth surfaces, and reduce their capacity to hold further plaque. The interdental surfaces are smoothed with fine linen polishing strips and dental floss coated in polishing paste. Finally, all the tooth surfaces are polished with a polishing paste using engine-driven rubber polishing cups and bristle brushes. A special handpiece should be used for polishing because the paste gets into the handpiece head and rapidly wears the moving parts spoiling them for accurate conservation work.

After a further period of oral hygiene, carried out by the patient at home, considerable improvement in the gingival condition is the usual result and then a further assessment can be made of the gingival contours and pockets to decide if surgery is indicated.

Gingival surgery

In suitable cases where the patient's co-operation, plaque control and interest is assured, moderate pockets can be eliminated surgically and the gingival contours can also be reshaped.

Surgery is carried out in stages so that the patient has only one side of the mouth operated upon at a time and can use the other comfortably during the healing stage.

Gingivectomy. Under anaesthesia the depths of the pockets in the operation site are marked (with the pocket-measuring forceps that punch through the pocket wall) to the level of the existing gingival attachment to the tooth. The unattached gingival tissue is then cut away by the use of specially angled gingivectomy knives (Fig. 11/2), e.g. Blake's Universal knife in which the tip of a Swann Morton scalpel blade is firmly held, or the Fish knives. The incision is carried along so that all the tissue is removed in one piece and afterwards any small tags remaining are carefully eliminated with further cautery or fine scissors. During the operation as in other forms of oral surgery, the DSA must work in close attendance using the sucker to keep the field free of saliva and blood.

The wound is dressed with an antiseptic paste such as Coe-Pak or other proprietary periodontal pack material. The pack is applied to the wound from both the lingual and buccal or labial surface and pressed and moulded firmly into place.

Flap operations. These are carried out when it is necessary to gain access to the pockets and the underlying bone, e.g. where bone defects exist as a result of periodontal disease and these have to be curetted (scraped) free of chronic infective products and granulation tissue to aid healing. When necessary the bone can be shaped and contoured with chisels or large sterile burs and diamond stones under a cooling stream of saline solution.

The planned flap incision is made with a sharp scalpel with a view to

145

GINGIVECTOMY INSTRUMENTS

Blake's universal

Pocket measuring probes

Fish

Fig. 11/2 Gingivectomy knives

removing the epithelial lining of the pocket, and the tissue reflected from the bone with a periosteal elevator. All the undesirable material and calculus is removed, the surfaces of the teeth planed smooth. Then the flap is replaced and sutured into position. The operation area is further protected with an antiseptic dressing pack.

After care. During the healing period, the patient is instructed to avoid eating on the operated side or disturbing the pack in any way. After about seven days, the pack and sutures may be removed in the surgery and the patient must then keep the area clean with a soft toothbrush, and an antiseptic mouthwash such as chlorhexidine solution up to 0.1%. As the area heals the patient can begin to brush the teeth and gingivae more vigorously each day and change to a medium toothbrush after about two to three weeks.

Functional abnormalities

In some cases the periodontal condition is aggravated by excessive occlusal pressures upon teeth due to malposition of a single tooth, malocclusion, premature loss of other teeth in the region, unopposed teeth, poor restorations, ill-fitting dentures or other appliances and nervous habits such as tooth-grinding (*bruxism*).

The occlusion is studied with the aid of models and by using articulating paper in the mouth to indicate points of contact. Treatment may be by selectively grinding away and reshaping certain teeth, by recontouring or replacing existing restorations, by remaking existing dentures or providing them for the first time so that they stabilise and support existing teeth. The effects of bruxism can be reduced by constructing a soft plastic bite guard, covering the occlusal surface of one jaw, to be worn by the patient at night.

In some cases, loosened teeth can be helped to survive occlusal pressures if they are splinted by a removable or fixed metal appliance to groups of healthy strong teeth elsewhere in the arch. Usually such matters are considered prior to the surgical phase.

Maintenance and prevention

Once the patient's course of treatment has been completed and his periodontal problem has been resolved as far as possible, it is vital that he is taught and maintains a high standard of oral hygiene (see page 200, Chapter 17) and returns regularly for thorough scaling and check-up. Should a relapse occur the patient may once again be unable to detect it himself.

SPECIFIC INFLAMMATORY CONDITIONS

Acute ulcerative gingivitis (Vincent's disease)

The exact cause of this disease is obscure, but it always occurs in association with specific organisms: *B. fusiformis*, a non-motile, thin, curved organism with tapering ends, and *Borellia vincenti*, a motile spirochaete. It is usually found in people of poor dental health, perhaps with a lowered general resistance to infection.

The onset of infection is sudden. Painful ragged ulcers occur locally on the interdental papillae and may spread quickly to affect the whole mouth and throat. There is a typical bad odour from the mouth, the temperature rises and the lymph nodes in the region are enlarged. The patient feels unwell and the appetite is lost.

Treatment. The mouth is gently cleansed with 10 volume hydrogen peroxide and peroxide mouthwashes are prescribed. At the same time a course of an antibiotic, e.g. penicillin, is given. Metronidazole (Flagyl) is also used for oral Vincent's infection. If necessary, investigation into the patient's general health is initiated. During the acute stage of the disease there is gross sepsis in the mouth and the patient should take common sense precautions to avoid contaminating his environment, e.g. in the preparation of food. He should also throw away his old tooth brush and obtain a new one. When the acute stage has subsided attention should be given to necessary thorough scaling and other periodontal treatment, oral hygiene and general health and dietary considerations.

Acute herpetic stomatitis

This is a virus infection usually first affecting children under the age of six, and thought to be transmitted by direct contact when the virus gains access to the underlying tissues through a small breach in the epithelium of the mouth. (Stomatitis means inflammation of the mouth.)

Small vesicles or blisters develop on the oral mucosa or lips and then burst leaving an open, painful ulcer which rapidly becomes secondarily infected by other organisms. During an attack the temperature rises, the appetite falls and small children are distressed and unwell. The ulcers begin to heal in about seven days and are generally completely healed in 14 days. The herpes virus remains dormant in the healed tissues and can be reactivated in later years by changes in the local tissue environment, e.g. 'cold sores' on the lips.

Treatment. The acute condition is treated by a general antibiotic, e.g. tetracycline, to combat the secondary infection and by the topical application of anaesthetic and antiseptic ointments to the ulcerated areas to reduce pain. Small children must be encouraged to drink fluids and may be coaxed to eat ice cream and bland non-spiced foods.

Pericoronitis

This is inflammation around an erupting tooth, generally a third molar, caused by eruption irritation, pressure on the overlying mucosa from the opposing tooth, food stagnation and secondary infection. The pain and discomfort is considerable and the patient may have swollen lymph nodes and find it difficult to open the mouth, *trismus*.

Treatment. This consists in raising the oral hygiene standards, the use of antiseptic mouthwashes, giving antibiotics if necessary and the removal of impacted teeth. In the acute stage extraction of the opposing tooth may be necessary.

Periodontal abscess

This is an abscess caused by spread of infection and destruction of tissue lateral to a tooth and deep in the periodontal tissues. Pus collects under pressure and there is localised painful swelling and inflammation below the gingival level. This condition must be differentiated from an apical abscess in which the infection arises as a result of a dead pulp.

Treatment. This is by drainage via the gingival crevice and/or incision of the abscess, hot saline mouthwashes and, where indicated by the patient's general condition, with general antibiotics. Extraction of the tooth may be necessary in some cases.

Thrush

This is a fungus infection of the mucous membrane of the mouth by a yeast *Candida albicans*. It is commonest in infants but is found occasionally in adults. It is due to a change in the balance of the oral bacteria brought about by unclean conditions, e.g. unsterilised feeding bottles and teats or dirty dentures, poor health or occasionally as the result of prolonged antibiotic or other therapy. It can affect all parts of the oral mucosa, but is more commonly found on the cheeks and tongue. It occurs as creamy-white patches which can be wiped off leaving a reddened area of mucosa.

Treatment. Attention must be paid to the causative factors and fungicidal drugs such as nystatin applied to the lesions.

Chapter Twelve

ANAESTHESIA

Anaesthesia is the loss of feeling or sensation in some part of the body due to a nervous lesion, anaesthetic agent or loss of consciousness. In surgery it is the term commonly used to denote loss of pain sensation produced in order that painful operations on the body can be performed. Anaesthetics are the drugs or chemical agents used to produce anaesthesia.

Local anaesthetics
These stop sensory nerve conduction by causing a reversible block to conduction along the nerve fibre and thus prevent sensation in a limited part of the body adjacent to the site of their injection or application, without loss of consciousness. (Note that some authorities prefer to use the term *analgesia* to describe this condition more precisely, for although pain sensation is eliminated some sense of pressure may remain. This descriptive precision in defining the two closely similar conditions is not yet universally used throughout the dental profession, but it is important to recognise the difference.) Topical or surface anaesthesia is a form of local anaesthesia produced by the application of a suitable agent to the surface of the skin or mucous membrane.

Regional anaesthesia
This is also called nerve block and is produced when a local anaesthetic drug is injected into the neighbourhood of a selected sensory nerve to block nerve conduction from a region of the body.

Relative analgesia
This is a method of inhalation sedation and analgesia produced by the administration of low concentrations of nitrous oxide to patients who remain conscious.

General anaesthesia
This is when drugs are given before and during surgical procedures to produce a state of unconsciousness and loss of painful sensations and also

to induce muscle relaxation. General anaesthetic agents are usually administered by allowing the patient to breathe in gases and vapours (inhalation anaesthesia) or by injection of a solution of the drug into a vein (intravenous anaesthesia).

INDICATIONS AND CHOICE

Anaesthetic drugs must not be given without careful consideration of the need for anaesthesia and the patient's condition on *every* occasion. All anaesthesia is an abnormal state produced with some degree of risk, however small, and should only be given when the relief more than compensates for the poisonous effect.

The pre-operative assessment of the patient will include consideration of fitness for operation, age, weight, the general health with particular reference to the cardiovascular, respiratory and central nervous systems and finally the emotional condition and the need for pre-operative sedation.

The type of anaesthetic used is dictated by the region, duration, noise and difficulty of the operation as well as the presence of infection and the patient's preference.

Local or regional anaesthesia. This is usually indicated for routine dental procedures frequently repeated (such as a course of conservation treatment), within limited areas and where there is no local infection that would be dispersed into the tissues by injection. It is also useful when the patient is unfit for general anaesthesia, e.g. in respiratory disorders.

Topical anaesthesia. This can be used in the mouth prior to local anaesthetic injection or on its own to assist surface procedures, e.g. deep scaling, fitting matrix bands, to prevent 'gagging' during impression taking and in treatment of painful ulcers.

Relative analgesia. This is used to alleviate fear and improve patient co-operation. There is a certain extent of analgesia, but pain is further controlled by the use of local anaesthetic agents.

General anaesthesia. This is indicated for operation in more than one quadrant of the mouth at once, in the presence of infection at the operation site (e.g. dental abscess) and for very young children or apprehensive or mentally handicapped patients of all ages. Many dental procedures are of short duration and can be carried out under general anaesthesia in the dental surgery; for longer operations, extensive surgery requiring endotracheal intubation or ill-health, the patient should be admitted to hospital.

LOCAL ANAESTHESIA

Local anaesthetic agents are active within five minutes of administration and their effect usually lasts about an hour. The duration of action of injected local anaesthetic drugs is increased if adrenaline is added to the solution to cause local vasoconstriction. Most local anaesthetic solutions contain the agent, adrenaline (or some other vasoconstricting drug), a trace of antiseptic and saline carefully balanced to prevent irritation of the tissues. Adrenaline is contra-indicated in cardiovascular disease and certain medical conditions.

Lignocaine hydrochloride (Xylocaine) is used in a 1% solution with adrenaline, producing extensive profound and prolonged anaesthesia. Lignocaine is also a very effective topical anaesthetic agent used in an ointment containing five per cent of the drug in a pleasantly flavoured base and in 4% sprays or solutions.

Prilocaine hydrochloride (Citanest) is a local anaesthetic of low toxicity which is similar to lignocaine. Its quick onset and prolonged action requires less vasoconstriction. It is used in 4% solution plain, or in 3% solution with felypressin as a vasoconstrictor. It may be given to patients whose medical condition contra-indicates adrenaline, e.g. those with heart or high blood pressure (hypertension) problems.

ADMINISTRATION

Topical anaesthetic agents. These are conveyed by a pledget of cotton-wool or a spray to the dried mucosal surface of the mouth. Their action is complete in two to five minutes and reduced if saliva washes the drug away prematurely.

Local anaesthetic solutions. These are injected with a syringe, commonly a dental cartridge syringe. The dental cartridge consists of 2ml of sterile local anaesthetic solution contained in a glass tube sealed at each end and it should remain in its sealed, sterile package until it is required. The cartridge is loaded into the sterile metal syringe framework where the syringe piston comes in contact with the rubber bung in the end of the glass tube. A sterile double-ended hypodermic needle attached to the other end of the syringe perforates the cap of the sealed tube so that pressure on the piston causes the solution to be expelled through the hollow needle. Needles are supplied in gamma-ray sterilised plastic containers. Needles should only be used on one occasion to eliminate the risk of cross-infection.

Before a patient is given a local anaesthetic a check should be made to ensure that they *have* eaten recently and if not, they should be given a glucose drink, for a low blood sugar increases any tendency to faint after injection. The patient should always be reassured and everything done to allay his apprehension prior to an injection.

Injection Techniques (Table 1)

Table 1 Local anaesthesia for teeth

	Teeth and associated tissues	Nerve supply	Injections used
87 | 78	Pulps, roots and perio- dontal structures Alveolar bone Buccal mucoperiosteum (gum)	Posterior superior alveolar nerve	Buccal infiltration by the tooth
	Palatal mucoperiosteum	Greater palatine nerve	Palatal infiltration by the tooth
6 | 6	Pulps, roots and perio- dontal structures Alveolar bone Buccal mucoperiosteum Palatal mucoperiosteum	Posterior and middle superior alveolar nerves Greater palatal nerve	Buccal infiltration by the tooth Palatal infiltration by the tooth
54 | 45	Pulps, both roots and periodontal structures Alveolar bone Buccal mucoperiosteum Palatal mucoperiosteum	Posterior and middle superior alveolar nerves Greater palatine nerve	Buccal infiltration opposite apex Palatal infiltration at level of apex
321 | 123	Pulps, roots and perio- dontal structures Alveolar bone Buccal mucoperiosteum Palatal mucoperiosteum	Anterior superior alveolar nerve Labial branches of infra-orbital nerve Long sphenopalatine nerve Long sphenopalatine nerve	Labial infiltration at level of apex Palatal infiltration
8-4 | 4-8	Pulps, roots and perio- dontal structures Alveolar bone Buccal mucoperiosteum Lingual mucoperiosteum	Inferior dental nerve Buccal nerve Mental nerve Lingual nerve	Inferior dental nerve block which also in- cludes lingual nerve block Buccal infiltration by side of tooth Lingual nerve block
3-1 | 1-3	Pulps, roots and perio- dontal structures Alveolar bone Labial mucoperiosteum Lingual mucoperiosteum	Incisive branch of in- ferior dental nerve Mental nerve Lingual nerve	Labial infiltration at the apex Lingual infiltration at the apex Jointly with labial infiltration Lingual infiltration at apex

Infiltration
The tip of the hypodermic needle penetrates the surface mucosa and the solution is injected slowly to allow it to diffuse into the deeper tissues.

All upper permanent teeth, lower incisors and canines and all primary teeth and their associated soft tissues and bone can be anaesthetised by infiltrating the solution over the apex of the tooth on both sides of the alveolus. Smaller quantities are used for children.

Inferior dental nerve block
This requires a long needle of larger diameter than that used for infiltration anaesthesia. With the patient's mouth wide open, the needle penetrates the mucosa behind the mandibular third molar region and slightly above the occlusal plane with the barrel of the syringe over the premolar region on the opposite side of the mandible. The needle is advanced along the inner surface of the ramus of the mandible until the tip lies next to the inferior dental and lingual nerves before the solution is slowly injected. This will anaesthetise the whole area served by these two nerves, including the pulps of the premolar and molar teeth and the lingual mucosa on that side. The patient will also be aware of a loss of sensation in the lower lip on the injected side. A further infiltration injection on the buccal aspect of these teeth will act upon the long buccal nerve serving the buccal mucosa and complete the anaesthesia required for extractions in the region.

Complications
Injection of the wrong drug. Always double-check the contents of the syringe with the dental surgeon.

Patient faints or collapses. See section on Emergencies, page 212.

Damage to the anaesthetised parts. Always manipulate or retract anaesthetised regions with care and gentleness. Warn the patient not to eat or smoke before the anaesthetic has worn off completely, and to avoid very hot drinks.

Out-of-date drugs. Never use anaesthetic solution that has become discoloured for it may be less potent, irritant or contaminated.

GENERAL ANAESTHESIA

The ideal general anaesthetic agent must be reversible, controllable, predictable, safe and have minimal side-effects. Many different drugs and techniques are used in dental surgery and the DSA should be well-rehearsed in her duties by the other members of the team before she assists with any case treated under general anaesthesia.

Inhalation anaesthesia

Nitrous oxide (dental gas) is a colourless, non-inflammable gas supplied in metal cylinders. It is the safest general anaesthetic agent if used correctly and allows quick recovery. In use it requires a marked reduction of the patient's circulating oxygen level and can be used alone only for very brief operations. In resistant patients other stronger anaesthetic agents have to be added to nitrous oxide to allow increased oxygen to be given if an operation lasts more than two minutes.

Halothane (Fluothane) is a colourless, volatile, non-inflammable liquid. It is a widely used agent, non-irritant, pleasant to inhale and with a low incidence of postoperative sickness. It is used in short procedures requiring rapid recovery, and may be combined with nitrous oxide and oxygen for dental anaesthesia. It can affect the heart rate and cause a fall in blood pressure during anaesthesia. It should not be used more than once every four to six months for a particular patient or it may cause liver function problems or jaundice. The dental team must make sure that there is adequate ventilation in the surgery when halothane is used, or they may suffer these cumulative effects themselves.

Trichloroethylene (Trilene) is a volatile, blue-dyed, non-inflammable liquid that can decompose to a poisonous gas if heated or if it comes into contact with strong alkalis in a closed-circuit anaesthetic apparatus. Its vapours are generally mixed with nitrous oxide and oxygen for dental anaesthesia. Disadvantages with its use are that recovery is often delayed, and postoperative vomiting occurs frequently.

Apparatus

The *inhalation anaesthetic apparatus* usually supports several *gas and oxygen cylinders* (which must be labelled 'Full' or 'In Use' so that they never run out without warning) whose flow passes through *pressure-reducing valves* and *flow controls* and is monitored by *flow meters* as it passes through flexible tubing to the patient. The flow can be diverted through *vapourising bottles* in order to take up volatile agents and a balloon-like *breathing bag* is included in the stream. The gases and vapours are delivered for the patient to inhale them via a *nose-* or *face-piece* (mask) and breathed out again through an *expiration valve* attached to it.

The *relative analgesia apparatus* is very similar but with two important differences: (1) the apparatus is pre-set so that it will not deliver less than 21% oxygen, and has a device that cuts off the nitrous oxide flow if the oxygen runs out; and (2) there is no provision for adding any other volatile agent to the mixture. The apparatus cannot produce anaesthesia.

Relative analgesia (Fig. 12/1)

Low concentrations of nitrous oxide in oxygen are given by inhalation to patients who remain conscious. The amount of nitrous oxide administered can be controlled within fine limits to suit a particular patient's needs. The gases may be given by the operator because of the high safety factors built

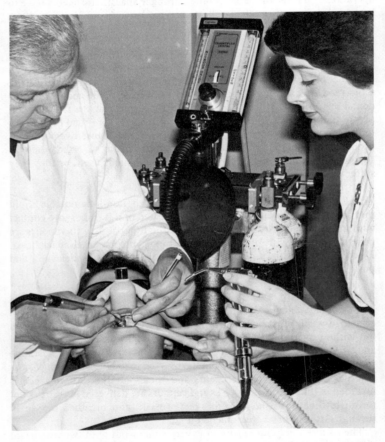

Fig. 12/1 Cavity preparation under relative analgesia. The DSA uses the high-speed suction tip to evacuate the handpiece water spray residue and saliva

into the apparatus. (This is the only circumstance where an anaesthetic agent may be administered to the patient by the operator. The use of general anaesthesia requires single minded constant attention to the patient's condition.) In addition all accepted measures for the management of emergencies must be available.

STAGES OF ANAESTHESIA

As the anaesthetic agent is taken in the patient passes through a sequence of stages of anaesthesia.

Stage 1: Analgesia (progressive loss of sensation to painful stimuli).

State 2: Delirium (unconscious, but reacts to stimuli such as noise).

Stage 3: Unconscious (with muscular relaxation – surgical anaesthesia).

Stage 4: Respiratory paralysis (the patient can only be kept alive by artificial respiration).

The anaesthetist can judge the stage at which the patient is being maintained by attention to such things as the patient's respiration rate, the skin colour, the eyes and so on. Oxygen and stimulant drugs should be available whenever a general anaesthetic is given.

INHALATION ANAESTHESIA

Preparation of the patient

The anaesthetist will check that the apparatus is switched on and in working order. He may need assistance from the DSA with regard to changing empty gas cylinders for full ones.

The patient should have signed his consent form for being given an anaesthetic. A parent must sign for a child under 16 years. He must *not* have taken food or drink for at least four hours before receiving a general anaesthetic to avoid the danger of inhaling vomit while unconscious. He should visit the toilet before going into the surgery.

The patient's identity is confirmed so that the correct records and radiographs are available. After the anaesthetist has examined him, the patient is seated in the chair, his collar and any other tight clothing that might impede respiration is loosened, any dentures are removed. In most cases a restraining strap is fastened round his waist as a seat belt and he is asked to interlock the fingers of each hand before the all-enveloping bib is put over him. The dental surgeon may again ask the patient his name, and briefly examines the teeth to be extracted and places a mouth prop in position unless the anaesthetist would prefer the prop at a later stage.

THE OPERATION

The operating light is turned off and the anaesthetist starts to administer the anaesthetic. Strict silence is observed in the room during this induction period. The DSA must be prepared with all the instruments required, but must also pay attention to the anaesthetist. When anaesthesia is achieved the DSA must switch on the operating light while the dental surgeon packs off the patient's mouth with a long gauze swab leaving the nasopharynx free for respiration. The DSA will then assist as required, this may include passing instruments, retracting and using a sucker tube. If the operation switches from one side of the mouth to the other the prop has to be changed over with the help of an expanding Mason's gag to hold the jaws open. The dental surgeon will remove the pack and the prop at the end of the operation. The anaesthetist will support the patient's head and check the airway.

POSTOPERATIVE CARE

When the operation ends the DSA will remain with the patient during the first recovery period with a kidney dish to hand for him to spit into or in case of vomiting. At no time whatsoever during the recovery stage should the unconscious patient be left unaccompanied. As consciousness returns a few soothing words will help the patient to re-orientate himself. Unless a trolley is available the patient may have to be assisted by two people to the recovery room to lie down for a while before going home, but nothing should be done to make him feel rushed at this stage of recovery.

The surgeon must satisfy himself that all the bleeding has stopped and the patient is physically fit to be discharged, before he can be allowed to leave.

Complications

Prolonged general anaesthesia with the unconscious patient in an upright position is ill-advised, because a fall in blood pressure may result in poor circulation and oxygen deprivation to the head and the risk of brain damage.

With a totally unconscious patient under a short-acting, yet potent, anaesthetic undergoing an operation in the region of the airway extreme vigilance is required to prevent any injury or untoward reaction. He must never be left alone. His position in the chair must remain satisfactory to avoid twisting his arms; he must be protected from injury by hot instruments, etc; his airway must be maintained clear and protected from foreign matter such as blood, vomit, pack or tooth. Where the patient leaves the surgery on a trolley and is still unconscious, he should be placed on his side and the airway protected by supporting the chin well forward as directed by the anaesthetist.

Following a general anaesthetic the patient should be escorted home by a responsible adult and forbidden to drive a car or work machinery for the rest of that day.

INTRAVENOUS ANAESTHESIA

An intravenous anaesthetic agent can be administered as a basal anaesthetic and followed up immediately by an inhalation anaesthetic in cases of difficult induction or fear of 'the mask'. They may also be used safely and effectively to produce a condition just short of surgical anaesthesia that is satisfactory for extraction or conservation of teeth. All intravenous methods should only be used by experienced skilled anaesthetists with full facilities and competence to deal with respiratory or cardiac complications. These drugs must not be given in certain medical conditions, e.g. liver disease.

Thiopentone sodium (Pentothal) is a yellow-white powder that is soluble in water. Given intravenously in a 2.5% freshly made-up solution it produces rapid anaesthesia which can be prolonged by further small doses at intervals. Recovery is fairly rapid.

Other intravenous anaesthetic agents include *methohexitone sodium* (Brietal Sodium) and *propanidid* (Epontol) both of which allow a more rapid final recovery. *Diazepam* is sometimes used to produce sedation and amnesia.

Preparation of the patient

This is the same as for an inhalation anaesthetic. The patient then lies down on his back (supine) (an advantage because it maintains a good circulation to the brain at all times). One sleeve, generally the left, is rolled up to expose the arm. Gripping and compressing the arm above the elbow (by the DSA in most cases) will cause the veins on the forearm and hand to stand out so that the anaesthetist can select and penetrate an appropriate vessel with the hypodermic needle. Before making an injection the skin is cleaned with an alcohol swab. As the drug is injected the compression is released. Where incremental doses are required arrangements are made to hold the needle in the vein by one of several methods and the patient's arm may be supported during the operation by strapping it to a rigid, gutter-like splint attached to the chair. The patient's eyes must be protected while he is supine. During the operation the airway must be protected from debris, blood and other fluids by the use of absorbent packs and high-velocity suction. For in-patients in hospital this is made more certain when an endotracheal tube is passed into the trachea and the throat packed off by the anaesthetist. A laryngoscope is used to allow the anaesthetist to see and illuminate the opening of the larynx.

At the end of the operation the anaesthetist will require the sucker with a wide-bore nozzle to complete this protection as the pack is removed.

Postoperative care

The patient is usually moved to the recovery room on a trolley as before. During the recovery period the patient is generally asked to lie on his side and spit out into a kidney dish. He should lie still in a quiet room until recovered enough to sit up comfortably. He should then sit in a chair for a further period before leaving the surgery. Once again he should only be discharged by the dental surgeon himself. As with inhalation anaesthesia he should be escorted home by another adult and forbidden to drive or operate machinery for the rest of that day.

Complications

These are rare if cases are carefully selected for this type of anaesthesia. The unconscious patient must be protected at all times as described in the section on inhalation anaesthesia. In the unlikely event of drug overdose the patient will require supportive measures by the anaesthetist to maintain the respiration and circulation until the drug effect wears off.

Intravenous injection must be carried out with care for if any of the drug is deposited in the tissues outside the vein it may cause postoperative pain and irritation in the region.

Chapter Thirteen

ORAL SURGERY

Oral surgery is the branch of surgery concerned with operations that are carried out on the jaws and associated soft tissues.

Treatment planning for surgery must be based on a thorough case history and diagnostic system with special attention to the patient's medical history and fitness for operation. Each operation should be planned carefully with step-by-step consideration of every stage including pre-medication (sedative or antibiotic), anaesthetic, operative technique, provisions for possible complications and postoperative care. Surgery must be carried out under strictly aseptic conditions to prevent wound cross-infection. The patient's records, including dental radiographs, must be available in the surgery for reference during any operation.

EXTRACTION OF TEETH

Extraction means the process of removing or drawing out a tooth from the mouth.

Teeth have to be extracted for many reasons including acute or chronic infection, grossly broken down teeth that cannot be conserved, impaction, supernumerary teeth, trauma and for orthodontic reasons.

Forceps (Figs. 13/1 and 13/2)

Dental forceps are designed to grip erupted teeth firmly at the neck. They are composed of handles, joint and beaks. They are made in a wide variety of shapes to fit the various anatomical contours of the teeth, to allow access to teeth in different regions of the mouth and also to suit the operator's personal preference.

Forcep extraction technique

The operator holds the forceps with the little finger between the handles to open the beaks. The blades of the beaks are inserted under the gingival margin and the forceps pressed up firmly before closing the handles to grip

UPPER ANTERIORS
AND ROOTS

Read pattern

UPPER BICUSPIDS
AND ROOTS

Split beak pattern

Left   Right

UPPER
MOLARS

UPPER ROOTS —   Bayonet pattern

Fig. 13/1 Forceps for the upper jaw

the tooth on cementum. The grip must be firm, but care must be taken not to crush the tooth and break it.

The tooth, forceps and arm are now a single lever used to enlarge the socket containing the tooth. The tooth is moved firmly in directions that will expand the socket and these forces vary according to the anatomy of the

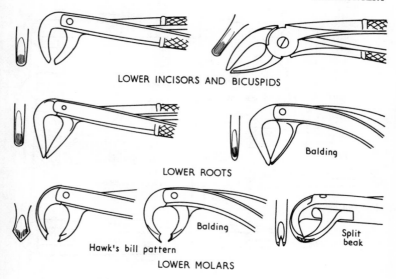

LOWER INCISORS AND BICUSPIDS

LOWER ROOTS

Balding

Hawk's bill pattern

Balding

Split beak

LOWER MOLARS

Fig. 13/2 Forceps for the lower jaw

tooth but are mainly in the direction of the thinner, weaker buccal plate. Some teeth, e.g. the upper central incisors, can be rotated. Finally, with the walls expanded and the periodontal attachment ruptured the tooth can be delivered from the socket. Note that teeth are never 'pulled out'.

When primary teeth are being extracted for a child great care must be taken not to damage or disturb the forming, unerupted permanent teeth beneath them.

The expanded walls of the socket should be closed again with finger and thumb pressure to reduce the possibility of post-extraction bleeding or pain and to promote the retention of a good blood clot that is the first stage of healing.

Elevators (Figs. 13/3 and 13/4)
Elevators are used to loosen and remove teeth which cannot be gripped by forceps, e.g. impacted teeth, to remove roots, to loosen teeth before application of forceps, to divide or split teeth or to remove bone between roots.

They are made in a very wide range of shapes both in blade, shank and handle.

Fig. 13/3 Apical and root elevators

The further division into 'Left' and 'Right' indicates the inclinations of the particular blades.

An elevator may be regarded first as a *wedge*, the sharp end being forced between the wall of the socket and the root, and then as a *lever* to move the root. They have to be used with great care because of the powerful leverage that can be generated. In some cases their action can be greatly assisted by the use of a bur to remove bone and allow their better access to the tooth.

SURGICAL EXTRACTIONS

In certain situations, e.g. broken roots or impacted teeth, an incision is made so that the overlying muco-periosteum can be reflected away in a flap from the region, and some overlying bone removed to allow better access to the tooth or root.

The flap incision is planned so that the reflected piece of muco-periosteum is large enough to allow adequate access to the underlying tissues. The flap must have a broad base to give it a good nerve and blood supply and to encourage postoperative healing. The incision must not sever important blood vessels or nerves in the region. The incision is made with a sharp *scalpel*, the bleeding sucked away immediately to allow good

Fig. 13/4 Root elevators

visibility. The flap is next stripped back with a *periosteal elevator* to uncover the bone and may then be held away from the operation site with a suitable *retractor*, e.g. the Austin retractor. Larger retractors may also be used to retract cheek, tongue, and so on.

Bone may be removed with suitable *surgical burs* or, under general anaesthesia, *chisels* and a *mallet* to allow access to the underlying tooth (Fig. 13/5). After the extraction is completed the margins of the bony wound may require smoothing with bone nibbling forceps or *rongeurs* and *files* before the wound is irrigated with sterile saline and closed. The flap is repositioned and sutured into place.

The sutures used intra-orally are generally of black braided silk. Occasionally resorbable catgut may be used because it does not have to be removed subsequently. Half-circle cutting edge needles are used in the

165

RONGEUR FORCEPS
Standard pattern

Coupland

OSSEOUS CHISELS

SURGICAL MALLET

AUSTIN RETRACTOR

FILE

PERIOSTEAL ELEVATORS

Fig. 13/5 Bone operating instruments

mouth and ready-threaded eyeless needles are obtainable in sterile packs.

The margin of the flap is gripped with toothed forceps, the curved needle is held in a pair of artery forceps (Spencer-Wells) or one of a range of special needle-holders. The needle is passed through the tissues, on either side of the incision line, the thread drawn after it and then knotted into place. Single or interrupted sutures are commonly used and after each knot the excess suture thread is cut away by the assistant with sharp scissors before the next suture is placed.

Sutures hold the tissues together, prevent haemorrhage, reduce infection and promote healing. Silk sutures have to be removed in four to seven days, generally a simple procedure not requiring anaesthesia.

SPECIAL OPERATIONS

Impacted teeth

Those teeth whose normal eruption into the mouth is prevented by adjacent teeth are described as impacted. The teeth most commonly squeezed out of the arch are third molars and canines which are much later in erupting than others alongside. They may sometimes be symptomless but more commonly give rise to pain (which may be referred to other parts of the face and head) or to local infections.

Lower third molars may lie impacted in a variety of inclinations; mesio-angular, disto-angular, vertical and horizontal and also at a variable depth from the occlusal plane. They thus present a wide range of difficulty and require expert assessment.

Broadly, the tooth is approached via a muco-periosteal flap and with the removal of overlying bone. In some cases a large tooth is deliberately divided with a bur or chisel, to allow it to be delivered through a small exit in two or three pieces.

Canine teeth may often be approached surgically from the palatal side of the arch.

Apicectomy (root amputation)

This is a method of dealing with infected tissue at the apex of a tooth that cannot be resolved by root canal therapy.

The tooth may be root-filled prior to operation or in some cases the open apex of the tooth is sealed with amalgam at the time of operation. A flap is made to expose bone over the affected apex and the overlying bone removed with burs. The apex is defined and cut off leaving at least two-thirds of the remaining root undisturbed. The diseased tissue is scraped away, *curetted*, with a spoon-shaped curette, the bone margins smoothed, irrigated with sterile saline and the flap sutured back into place.

Simple cysts

Again an overlying muco-periosteal flap is retracted and bone is removed to expose the cyst lining. Small cysts can be curetted away entirely, *enucleated*, and the cavity closed with the flap to heal normally. Large bony cysts may have to be allowed to collapse over a period by *marsupialising* them. The superficial wall of the cyst is cut away and the opening made to persist by inserting a suitable plug. Each day the pouch of the cyst cavity is washed clean and the plug replaced. Rapidly, over the course of weeks, quite large cyst cavities will collapse and fill up from the bottom with new bone.

Prosthetic preparation

A wide range of operations may be carried out to facilitate the construction of dentures. Bone and soft tissue contours of the ridges, bony swellings on the hard palate, and the depths of sulci can all be changed surgically. Where multiple extractions have been carried out, removal of inter-radicular bony septa and collapse of the labial walls of the sockets can overcome maxillary protrusion for example.

Dental implants. These are used occasionally and there are many techniques. For example, in two consecutive operations (the first for bone preparation and an impression) a prepared metal framework is placed in contact with the shaped bone of the ridge and the mucosa sewn back into place, leaving locating studs projecting through the tissues into the mouth. The denture superstructure is made to fit on these studs and gains considerable retention in this way.

Biopsy

The tissue to be examined is removed using a scalpel and toothed dissecting forceps and transferred to a screw-capped specimen bottle containing preservative solution such as formo-saline. The bottle must be clearly labelled and accompanied by a short history of the condition and instructions, when despatched to the laboratory. (Check with the pathology laboratory of the local hospital about special precautions to be taken if the specimens are to be sent to them by post.)

Abscess drainage

Occasionally an abscess is neglected or occurs so quickly that by the time the patient arrives at the dental surgery a considerable swelling has occurred. When necessary, in addition to antibiotic therapy and extraction or opening a tooth to drain via the root canal, the soft tissue swelling has to be incised to let out the accumulated pus.

Intra-oral incisions may be made into the centre of the abscess (where it 'points') with a scalpel. Though rarely necessary, extra-oral drainage is also carried out by incision, taking great care not to sever arteries or nerves and may be further assisted by blunt dissection with artery forceps. Extra-oral wounds should be covered with a dry dressing.

POSTOPERATIVE CARE

Haemorrhage

The patient should not be allowed to leave the surgery until all bleeding has ceased. He should be given careful instructions not to disturb the clot, not to use excessive mouthwashes or take very hot food or drinks and to avoid alcohol and excessive bodily activity for the next twenty-four hours. He should be advised how to apply haemostatic pressure to the wound by biting on a firm pad, e.g. a clean handkerchief, should any bleeding recur (see Chapter 18).

Swelling

Potential postoperative swelling of the soft tissues of the face and jaws may be reduced after extensive and prolonged surgery by the local application of cold. An ice bag or a rubber glove containing ice can be applied to the face for several minutes each hour as directed by the dental surgeon for the following twenty-four hours. Ice packs must be used with care to prevent skin damage occurring.

Pain

The patient should be given a supply of a mild analgesic drug such as aspirin or paracetamol for use should postoperative pain occur.

Infection

An aseptic technique should minimise this complication, but pre-and postoperative antibiotic therapy may be necessary in some cases. Healing may be promoted by the use of frequent hot saline mouthwashes after the first twenty-four hours.

Dry socket

A localised infection of alveolar bone (osteitis) following tooth extraction. This painful condition arises due to premature loss of blood clot, perhaps due to excessive mouth rinsing immediately after extraction. It is more common in the mandible. Treatment involves syringing the socket clean with saline and dressing it with zinc oxide/eugenol or a proprietary paste. The patient may also require antibiotics and analgesia.

Medication and anaesthetics

The patient should be made aware of the after-effects that any drugs and anaesthetic agents used may produce. Pre-medication usually causes

169

drowsiness, so the patient must be accompanied by a responsible adult, as must a patient who is to have a general anaesthetic. The patient must never be allowed to drive a car while under the influence of these drugs.

Anxiety
The patient must be told who to contact in an emergency should he become anxious about any postoperative aspect of the surgical treatment.

FRACTURES
Fractures of the jaws and the facial bones fall within the scope of oral surgery, but as a specialised field generally only dealt with in hospital. Many forms of fracture occur and each demands different details of treatment.

Broadly, fractured bones have to be replaced into their correct position, *reducing* the fracture, held firmly in place, *immobilisation*, for the required number of weeks, the patient's general health maintained, and swelling, infection and pain combated while healing takes place. After healing, the immobilisation or *fixation* is removed and the part *rehabilitated*.

Often the fractured segments of the jaws hold firm teeth and these can be fastened together and to the opposing teeth by wires or cast silver splints to immobilise the fracture. Where the angle of the fracture is not favourable for this form of immobilisation or no teeth exist on the fragments, the bones may be wired together directly and the fixation achieved by pins driven into the bone extra-orally and linked to each other by special screw brackets and bars perhaps extending to a firm anchorage in a plaster head cap or metal halo.

Great attention has to be paid to making up an interesting and nourishing semi-liquid diet for a patient whose jaws are immobilised.

Wider applications of oral surgery
The scope of oral surgery extends into and links up with the fields of general surgery in the treatment of tumours, extensive head and neck injuries, plastic surgery, and many dental techniques are of value in other fields, e.g. maxillo-facial prostheses.

Chapter Fourteen

PROSTHETICS

Prosthetic dentistry is that part of restorative dentistry concerned with the construction of removable appliances to replace lost teeth. These prosthetic appliances are called dentures. They are generally described by their extent, e.g. full dentures and partial dentures, and by the materials from which they are made, e.g. acrylic, gold, chrome-cobalt.

Although these appliances are made with extreme care, skill and ingenuity they can never be as satisfactory as sound natural teeth.

AIMS OF DENTURE CONSTRUCTION

1. To retain masticatory function.
2. To restore and maintain good appearance and prevent changes in facial contours and temporomandibular joint function due to reduced muscular activity or loss of bite height.
3. To maintain clear speech. The loss of teeth, particularly at the front of the mouth, can hamper the pronunciation of certain sounds.
4. To prevent overeruption of unopposed teeth, tilting of teeth adjacent to a space and the production of excessive strain on the periodontal structure of the remaining teeth.

A great many different techniques are used in making dentures, but only two basic methods can be described here as common examples.

CONSTRUCTION OF FULL DENTURES

Following the extraction of teeth, the sockets in the alveolus heal first by organisation of the blood clot into fibrous tissue and then by conversion of this to bone. The healed alveolar bone and its overlying tissues form a ridge. This ridge will be large and broad to begin with, but gradually over the years it will resorb and reduce in size. In extreme age, or in cases where there has been extensive bone destruction due to periodontal disease before the extractions, the ridge can become very thin and shallow and present little for a denture to be based upon.

Preliminary treatment plan
A careful case history and a complete survey of the edentulous (toothless) mouth is essential plus the study of any available pre-extraction records (models or photographs) or previous dentures.

First appointment. First impressions are taken of the upper ridge and hard palate and the lower ridge using impression compound in selected stock impression trays. The laboratory instructions should indicate which type of impression material will be used for the second working impressions.
Laboratory work. The first impressions are cast by vibrating a creamy mix of plaster of Paris into them. When this has set hard the trays and impression material are removed and any surplus plaster trimmed away neatly. These models are examined and the outlines of the denture-bearing areas are marked out in pencil. Special trays, made of plastic or shellac are constructed on these models with their margins contoured to include the denture-bearing areas.

Second appointment. The second more accurate working impressions are taken. The special trays are tried in the mouth and adjusted as necessary to avoid muscle attachments or overextension of the margins, with files, large burs and sandpaper. Additions to the tray margins may be made with a tracing stick compound if necessary before the impressions are taken in plaster impression paste or alginate. (Alginate impressions must not be allowed to dry out on their way to the laboratory.)
Laboratory work. The working impressions are cast in hard stone. The trays and impression materials are removed and the models trimmed. Wax *occlusion rims* are constructed on firm *base plates* of acrylic or heated moulded shellac material made to fit the denture-bearing areas.

Third appointment. The jaw relations are registered. The occlusion bite rims are tried in the mouth and the bases adjusted, if necessary, until they are a comfortable fit. The wax rims are then trimmed and contoured with a heated wax knife to indicate the amount of bulk required to support the upper lip, the occlusal plane and to register the correct amount of space between the jaws. The vertical relationship may be checked with a bite gauge or callipers to measure distances between the nose and chin both with the rims together and with the jaws in a relaxed position and the mouth empty. (These measurements are made according to certain conventions that will differentiate between the resting position and the functional position and require very careful judgement.) The rims are finally sealed together in the mouth with jaw registration paste in the retruded or 'central' jaw relationship, so that they may be reassembled in the correct position outside the mouth. The centre line, the resting lip line, the high lip line and the corners of the mouth are marked on the wax with the rims in position in the mouth. The make, colour, size and shape of the teeth to be used are considered and indicated on the laboratory instructions. (Among prosthetics specialists the old term 'taking the bite' is being superseded by the more precise term 'registering the centric jaw relationship' and 'bite blocks' are now called 'occlusion rims'.)

Laboratory work. The models are set on a mechanical reproduction of the jaw movement called an *articulator* in the position indicated by the bite. Individual acrylic or porcelain teeth are set up in pink wax mounted on base plates adapted to fit these models. Great care is taken to arrange the teeth to give a good appearance and the occlusion is checked in centric and functional positions by movement of the articulator mechanism. Finally the waxed-up model dentures are smoothed and contoured to the shape of the finished appliances.

Fourth appointment. The wax model dentures are tried in the mouth. They are cooled first in cold water so that they will not be distorted by the body heat. In the mouth they are checked for facial and lip appearance, for occlusion in centric and functional positions, for bite height and for size, length, arrangement and colour of the teeth. If all is well the patient is asked to check them visually in a hand mirror. Small adjustments of individual teeth can be made at the chairside, out of the mouth, by warming the wax with a hot wax knife and moving the tooth as required. More extensive alterations may mean that the work must be returned to the laboratory and a further re-try appointment made. When all is satisfactory, the final outlines of the dentures are drawn on the models in pencil, with special attention to all muscle attachments and the posterior palatal margin of the upper denture. Where a bony ridge is present that may be expected to cause the denture to rock, e.g. in the mid-line of the hard palate, a *relief area* is indicated in outline.

Laboratory work. The denture area is marked on the model with a pin-line scratched along the pencil line indications and the posterior palatal margin of the upper denture is cut widely into the model so that a ridge will be formed on the denture (the post-dam seal). Any relief area is covered with a thin layer of metal foil. This foil will be stripped away from the processed denture to leave a hollow in the fitting surface The wax dentures are sealed on to the stone models at their margins and the models, plus the wax and teeth are set into a sectional plaster mould constructed in a metal box (a dental flask) by pouring carefully separated sections of plaster over them. When the final mix of plaster has set, the flask is warmed in hot water until

173

the wax softens and then the sections of the flask can be separated so that one holds the artificial teeth firmly, the other the stone model while the walls record the contours of the rest of the denture shape. The wax can now be washed away with hot water. The cooled plaster is coated with a sodium alginate separating paint ('cold mould seal') carefully avoiding the teeth and then a fresh mix of soft acrylic dough is packed into the mould. The flask is reassembled and placed under pressure until all the excess acrylic is extruded and the flask closed firmly. The closed flask is clamped and heated in a water bath as necessary. When the acrylic has been processed (cured) and hardened the flask is cooled and then opened and the denture separated from the plaster mould. The surplus material at the edges of the denture is cut away as indicated by the original pin-lines and the cut surfaces smoothed with files, burs, stones and sandpaper. The dentures are finished and polished against revolving brushes, mops and felt wheels on a large lathe first using pumice and water followed by finer polishing agents such as whiting and water until the final high polish is achieved. The fitting surface is not polished.

Fifth appointment. The finished dentures are fitted. The upper denture is inserted first and checked for border extension, appearance and retention. Retention is achieved partly by border seal and partly by the close contact between the saliva-moistened fitting surfaces of the denture and the mucosa of the palate and ridge (in the same way that two flat glass slabs hold firmly together when their contacting surfaces are wet). This intimate contact may only develop properly when the denture has been worn for a few days. Next the lower denture is inserted and examined. The retention of the lower denture depends mainly on muscular control with the lips, cheeks and tongue and the elimination of any displacing forces as well as the wet contact of the fitting surface and mucosa. The occlusion is checked in centric and functional positions. If necessary a small amount of a gum denture fixative may be used to hold the dentures firmly and increase the patient's confidence. The patient now checks the appearance again in a hand mirror. The patient is shown how to remove and insert the dentures, told how to clean them and usually advised about how long to wear them each day. He is also recommended to eat carefully until the dentures are fully settled in and adjusted. They must certainly be worn for several hours immediately preceding the next follow-up appointment.

Sixth appointment. The patient returns after an interval of a few days for a check-up to allow the dental surgeon to hear and see how he is progressing with the dentures. The denture-bearing areas are examined for signs of inflammation or ulcers caused by excessive pressure points and the dentures eased and adjusted as necessary. The occlusion is also checked and adjusted. When all is well, the patient is asked to return if necessary for further small adjustments, but in any case to return in one year for re-assessment. All full dentures need check-ups and adjustments at intervals and it is unwise to neglect them indefinitely.

CONSTRUCTION OF PARTIAL DENTURES

Partial dentures are constructed to replace a missing tooth or group of teeth in a functional and aesthetic way. They take their support partly from the mucosa and partly from the remaining natural teeth by means of *clasps* (supporting arms attached to the denture and in contact with a natural tooth) and *occlusal rests* (rigid extensions lapping over the occlusal surfaces to resist occlusal pressure that could drive the denture hard against the underlying mucosa). Great care must be taken in their design and construction to avoid disrupting the natural occlusion, over-stressing the remaining teeth or causing damage to the oral mucosa and gingival margins.

Preliminary treatment plan. A case history and complete oral survey including radiographs of the remaining teeth are essential before deciding to construct a denture. Any necessary conservation and periodontal treatment must be completed before the working impressions are taken.

First appointment. First impressions of the upper and lower jaws are taken in selected stock trays using alginate, and a wax leaf occlusion registration

Fig. 14/1 Taking an impression. The DSA is mixing alginate impression material

175

made where possible (Fig. 14/1). The laboratory work-slip should indicate which material will be used for the second impression.

Laboratory work. The models are cast in plaster and special trays are constructed in plastic. (However if the dental surgeon has decided that stock tray impressions are adequate to finish the denture on, the models are cast in stone, occlusion rims are made on firm base plates and the case proceeds to 'Third Appointment'.)

Whenever possible the models are mounted on an articulator before the final design is made. The model is examined and *surveyed* to choose the best path of insertion, so that clasps can be put in the most effective positions around the teeth and any undercuts (the spaces beneath overhanging teeth or tissues when looked at from the chosen line of insertion) blocked out. Occlusal rests and clasps are planned so that when they are seated on the teeth they will not interfere with the occlusion in centric or functional positions.

Second appointment. The final design for the finished denture should be agreed at this stage in order that any adjustments to the natural teeth may be made by grinding before the second impressions are taken. Finally, the accurate working impressions are taken in the special trays using an elastic impression material such as alginate.

Laboratory work. The working models are cast in hard stone and wax occlusion blocks made on firm base plates. *Note:* Some partial denture cases have so few natural teeth missing that the models can be articulated without requiring an occlusion block, although most dental technicians would prefer to have a wax leaf occlusion registration even in such a case.

Third appointment. The occlusion is registered in the mouth by trimming and marking the occlusion blocks as necessary with a wax knife. The shade of the teeth is matched with a shade guide and this is sometimes very difficult for natural teeth are rarely all the same colour in one mouth as they vary in thickness, fillings, vitality, staining, and so on.

Laboratory work. If a metal base or 'skeleton' framework is to be used in the final denture it is now constructed in metal, e.g. a gold or chrome-cobalt casting. The metal clasps and rests are contoured and fitted to the teeth (in some cases the technician prefers to leave these small structures to be made in the finishing stage). Finally the whole structure is waxed up on a base that is removable from the model: artificial teeth, clasps, rests, skeleton, and prepared for a try-in.

Fourth appointment. The model denture is tried in the mouth and checked for design, occlusion and appearance and any small adjustments made. The patient also checks the appearance in a hand mirror. Large adjustments must be made in the laboratory and checked once more at a re-try appointment before proceeding to a finish.

Laboratory work. The denture is flasked, packed, processed and finished in a similar way to a full denture.

Fifth appointment. The denture is fitted, checked again for the design, occlusion, function and appearance and any small adjustments made at the chairside. The patient is shown how to remove and replace the denture, how to clean it and the natural teeth it comes in contact with, paying particular attention to the clasped teeth.

Sixth appointment. After a few days the denture is checked again at a follow-up appointment. Any occlusal high spots or points of excessive pressure on the mucosa are eased and any other small adjustments are made. When all is well the patient is asked to return if necessary for further small adjustments. The denture will be re-examined routinely at each regular six-monthly check-up in the future.

Repairs

If a denture breaks, commonly as a result of having been mishandled out of the mouth, the technician can usually join the pieces together and effect a repair. This is fairly simple in the case of a clean fracture of acrylic when the fragments can be accurately repositioned. When there is any doubt about the positions of the pieces, or if a fragment or tooth is lost, a new impression will be required and sometimes an occlusion record of the opposing teeth. When metal has broken, the problem is more complex because it may mean removing the acrylic and teeth from a skeleton denture so that the fracture may be repaired by soldering. Close liaison with the technician is necessary to confirm the kind of impression and occlusal records he will require for a particular case.

Relines

Full dentures will gradually loosen because of ridge resorption after they have been worn for a few years, although remaining otherwise satisfactory. New fitting surfaces may be processed into them by a relining technique.

The denture is prepared for relining by trimming flanges and any undercuts and slightly roughening the fitting surface. A zinc oxide impression paste is applied thinly to the fitting surface and the denture carefully positioned in the mouth. The opposing denture is put in the mouth and the patient instructed to close firmly so that the impression is held accurately in position and the vertical jaw relationship is not 'raised'. The peripheral margins are contoured by protruding and retracting the lips. When the paste has set, the denture and the impression it contains is sent to the laboratory. The technician casts a model and plaster overbite, cuts away the whole of the old fitting surface and processes a new one in its place. When finished and polished the result is a well-fitting appliance with the same appearance and occlusion as before.

SPECIAL APPLIANCES

Immediate dentures. These are made on models of the mouth made before the teeth are extracted. The teeth to be lost are cut away from the model during the final stages of making the denture and their acrylic replacements waxed into place. At the time of extractions, the empty sockets are immediately covered with the new denture so that the patient is at no time left without teeth. Normal healing takes place under the denture. This method is used commonly to replace anterior teeth, particularly for people who have to appear before the public or who would be embarrassed to be without teeth until healing had taken place. Immediate dentures usually require relining after about six months because of the post-extraction ridge shrinkage that normally occurs during this period.

Overlays. In certain circumstances, e.g. temporomandibular joint disturbances, overlays are constructed that cover all the occlusal surfaces of the teeth in one jaw to raise the jaw relationship to a new functional level.

Obturators. When a patient has a defective palate due to congenital cleft palate, or as a result of surgery or an accident, an obturator ('stopper') based on a denture can be constructed to seal the defect, assist speech and prevent food and liquids from leaking from the mouth to the nose. Care must be taken during the impression stage to prevent the material from passing up into the nose and perhaps getting impacted there.

Maxillo-facial prostheses. Where a patient has suffered a loss of parts of the jaws, lips, nose or other parts of the face as a result of disease, injury or surgery and it is not possible to restore the parts by plastic surgery, the specialist dental team may be called in to use dental techniques and materials to make an artificial restoration of the lost tissue. These appliances can be made to look very realistic even at close quarters. This is difficult but rewarding work because successful results will allow such patients to return to normal lives in the community.

IMPRESSION MATERIALS

Impression materials are either rigid or elastic in character and may be thermoplastic or non-reversible.

178

Thermoplastic materials
Impression compound. A material made up of waxes, gums, resins and inert mineral fillers which is reversibly soft and plastic when heated and hard and rigid upon cooling. Pieces of the composition are placed in a water bath at 55 to 60°C until softened. A quantity is worked and moulded into a soft ball with the fingers, transferred to a dry metal impression tray and moulded to fit it. Any excess material is pulled off at the edge of the tray. The surface of the composition is warmed briefly over a clean flame to soften and smooth the surface and the tray and its contents are then dipped into the hot water to temper the material and ensure that no part remains flame-heated enough to burn the patient's mouth. The tray and composition is seated in place in the mouth and the cheeks, lips and tongue moved to mould the margins accurately. The impression is supported in position until the composition is cooled sufficiently to remove it from the mouth without distorting it.

Tracing stick is a composition that is softer at lower temperatures than ordinary impression composition and in pencil-thick rods may be flame heated and used to make corrective or tissue-compressing additions to larger previous composition impressions or special trays.

Non-reversible materials
Plaster of Paris. This is dehydrated calcium sulphate and is a white, odourless and tasteless powder which can take up moisture from the air. When mixed to a smooth paste with water it sets in about three minutes and hardens in 15 to 20 minutes It can be used as a rigid impression material, as well as for the construction of models and as an ingredient of investment material in casting metals. For impressions it is mixed with an anti-expansion solution, which also accelerates the setting time, containing measured amounts of salts such as potassium sulphate and borax.

A quantity of anti-expansion solution is placed in a clean rubber bowl, fine plaster of Paris powder is sprinkled evenly over the surface and allowed to soak in until a fine dry layer lies on the top. After 20 seconds the mixture is carefully spatulated, to avoid air bubbles, for 30 to 40 seconds and vibrated by banging the bowl down once or twice to cause any air bubbles that might have been produced to rise and be eliminated from the mix. The special impression tray is then filled with the mix and inserted into the mouth as the plaster starts to thicken. The setting time, usually one and a half to two minutes in the mouth, is judged by observing the condition of the plaster remaining in the bowl. If the plaster breaks on removing the impression from the mouth, the fractures are clean and sharp and the pieces are easily reassembled before the impression is cast. A separating medium such as soap solution must be applied to the surface of the impression before casting it or the plaster will unite with the model material.

Commercially available impression plasters include the anti-expansion salts with the plaster in the container, and need only be mixed with water.

Impression paste. This material is rigid in character and cannot reproduce extensive undercuts. It may be used as a relining impression material and also in special trays to give an accurate working impression for an edentulous case.

Two pastes are provided, one containing, for example, oil of cloves and a resin and the other zinc oxide powder, lanolin and water. Equal quantities of the two pastes are measured out by length on a disposable mixing paper, mixing pad or a thin card and thoroughly spatulated to a creamy homogeneous consistency. White petroleum jelly is smeared on the patient's lips to prevent the paste from sticking to the skin. The paste is spread evenly over the impression surface of the tray or denture and inserted into the mouth. After about four to five minutes, when the material has hardened, the impression is removed from the mouth and inspected. Small deficiencies or air blows in the impression can be corrected by adding further small amounts of freshly mixed paste and replacing the impression in the mouth for a further period.

Alginates. These elastic, jelly-like materials, which contain some 20 per cent of inert filler, are non-reversible and can be used to reproduce undercut areas of teeth and ridge in the mouth. The gel is formed as a result of chemical action by combining a calcium salt with a solution of sodium or potassium alginate. The calcium gradually replaces the sodium and calcium alginate is precipitated in the form of an insoluble gel. When set these materials are not adhesive and must be held in the tray either mechanically, by allowing them to ooze through perforations in the tray, or by painting a sticky material on to the tray surface before loading it.

Carefully measured quantities of alginate powder and water must be used and the water must be at the correct temperature (20°C or in accordance with the manufacturer's instructions). The water is put into a rubber bowl, the powder added all at once and the materials mixed and spatulated thoroughly for some 30 seconds. The mix is loaded into the prepared tray, taking care not to overload it, and the tray positioned in the mouth. The material is allowed to set undisturbed for about three minutes. After removal from the mouth the material must not be allowed to dry out or the impression will become distorted. To prevent this the tray and its impression may be stored in a sealed container, such as a plastic bag, although it is better if these impressions are cast up immediately.

Synthetic rubber. See the section on indirect inlay impression technique for details of the use and mixing of this elastic, non-reversible material. (p.125)

DENTURE BASE MATERIAL

Acrylic resin (methyl methacrylate)

This popular thermoplastic denture base material is formed by the linking together of chemical molecules into chains (polymerisation) to form a solid material composed of microscopic tangled masses of threads. When heated the formed material may be softened, to harden again on cooling, but it is simpler to pack a mould with newly prepared material in dough form and allow it to polymerise to the new shape.

Acrylic resin denture base materials are supplied as a stable polymerised powder (polymer) and an unpolymerised volatile liquid (monomer). Plasticising agents and colouring materials have been added to these constituents to improve the workability and produce the required colour.

The powder and the liquid are mixed in the recommended proportions in a glass or pottery jar and, in a short time as the reaction begins, the monomer is itself converted to polymer and links the granules of the powder together. The damp sand-like mix becomes sticky and stringy and soon forms a plastic dough. This dough is rapidly packed into the prepared flask before it becomes rubbery and the flask is closed under pressure. The clamped flask and its contents are heated in boiling water to 'cure' the material for the recommended period until the conversion of the remaining free monomer to stable polymer has been completed and the denture can proceed to the next stage.

'Cold-cure' acrylic materials are available that also contain accelerating agents and these will set completely with minimal pressure and without the application of heat. They must be used with care or free monomer may persist in the material and act as an irritant to the oral mucosa.

All acrylic resins absorb water and contract if they are allowed to dry out. Thus acrylic dentures should be stored in cold water before the patient receives them and should be kept in water when they are not in use.

Acrylic is not very resistant to abrasives and dentures should only be cleaned by brushing with soap and water and by soaking stains off with a proprietary denture bath solution if they are to retain their high polish.

Chapter Fifteen

DENTISTRY FOR CHILDREN

Paedodontics or children's dentistry includes all aspects of child dental health up to the arbitrary age of thirteen years. It is mainly concerned with preventive dentistry, operative dentistry and orthodontics for this age-group and successful treatment procedures require some knowledge of basic child psychology.

The importance of child dental health cannot be overemphasised for the first steps in dental care and in planning and carrying out any necessary dental treatment will affect the child's dental condition and attitude to treatment for the rest of its life. Every other aspect of dentistry in later years can only be in a 'follow-up' capacity. Although this chapter is devoted to child management and operative treatment for children, remember that preventive dentistry is of prime importance at this age.

CHILD MANAGEMENT

A child's first attitude to dentistry will be copied from the parents and other members of the family who may themselves be apprehensive about dental treatment. Some parents are ignorant of the value of the primary teeth and regard them as trivial nuisances that should be extracted if they cause trouble. Sometimes reluctance to seek treatment means that a child's mouth is neglected until severe pain or infection occurs and the child's first introduction to dentistry is unavoidably unpleasant for him.

Importance of primary teeth

Parents must be made aware of the importance of maintaining the primary teeth in a healthy condition because:
1. They are necessary for proper mastication of a balanced diet during the child's important growing years.
2. They are part of the apparatus of speech and needed especially when the child is learning to speak.
3. They are required in the mouth to maintain space in the arch during growth of the jaws. Premature loss could aggravate possible crowding of

the permanent teeth and perhaps lead to the necessity for prolonged orthodontic treatment later.

4. The teeth play an important part in the child's appearance and their early loss may be bad for any child's self-confidence.

5. The extraction of teeth, no matter how skilfully carried out, is not a pleasant experience for a child, even if he is old enough to understand why it has to be done.

As they grow older children pass through a series of attitude changes, and it is helpful to be aware of them when the child is brought into the dental surgery.

Infant

A child's mouth plays a very important role in his general psychological make-up. At first a baby's mouth becomes a source of comfort and pleasure as he takes in milk and food to satisfy hunger pains and he gradually becomes aware of the different textures, temperatures and tastes. This connection between stomach, mouth, comfort and security becomes interwoven with many other basic themes but it always remains as a strong instinct in the subconscious. Any oral pain, discomfort or loss of teeth must therefore have a deep psychological effe   as well as that at the superficial physical level, especially in the young child who cannot understand why it has happened to him.

Pre-school child

Very young children often have regular sleeping periods during the afternoon and appointments should be made to avoid these times. Up to about two and a half years old the child is strongly dependent upon his mother or mother substitute and looks to her for signals about how to react to his surroundings. He will be more upset by being separated from her than by any treatment procedure and may react best sitting or even lying on her lap. From this age any repetitive sequence of events can be used to accustom him gradually to treatment because it makes the whole thing into a game. The 'T.S.D.' technique is useful: *Tell* the child what is to be done, 'I'm going to brush your teeth', *Show* him the brush, 'This is the brush I'm going to brush your teeth with', and *Do* brush his teeth, 'I'm brushing your teeth like this'.

At about two and a half years old, most children discover that they have a personality of their own which they assert by refusing to comply with simple direct commands. It is useless to ask for their direct co-operation, but various subterfuges can help in which the child is given an apparent choice of action, e.g. which of two burs should be used on his tooth, or whether he would like a warm or cold mouthwash. From this age children

183

are very susceptible to praise about their dress or some other external feature.

At three the child wants to help and be involved in every activity. Now he understands a larger range of words and can be controlled more easily with interesting conversation. However never let a young child discover too much about the workings of the fascinating dental equipment or he will use it as a delaying tactic and waste potential treatment time.

At four the child's self-confidence has usually expanded. He is very definite and vocal in his opinions and physically more active but is able to co-operate more readily and for longer periods. He responds to praise and being treated as a 'grown-up'. He is full of questions and these have to be answered during the continuation of treatment procedures or they become a delaying weapon. At this age a child will boast about his dental experiences later on, so make sure that his imagination has nothing unexplained to work on.

School child
At about five most children start school and this has the effect of suddenly expanding his social experience. He leaves the home environment for much of the day to become one of a large group and has to conform to new behaviour patterns, timetables and rivalries. He gets tired at the end of the day and should have morning appointments. He is more composed and able to accept prolonged dental procedures more easily. He becomes more mouth conscious at this time for he is starting to shed the first of the primary teeth.

From six to ten years the child goes through a more body-conscious stage in which he is more afraid of potential damage to his body than of separation from his parent. The dental drill, the injection needle, extractions, blood, and so on, are all particularly worrying at this age and their unavoidable presence has to be reduced to a minimum by careful technique and explanation.

Adolescence
Eleven- to thirteen-year-olds are going through the first stages of adolescence with its general unsettling effects on self-confidence and the ability to come to terms with changes in bodily function and mental attitudes. The physical appearance becomes of marked importance in most cases and treatment of the upper incisor teeth will carry great significance from now on. Young teenage boys who have previously been regular attenders go through a stage of regarding routine dental treatment as an unnecessary convention and begin to fail appointments. In doing this, psychologists believe that the boy is overlaying a deeper Freudian fear of bodily mutilation and loss of manhood.

Basic behaviour patterns

It appears that there are three main types of normal children who arrive in the dental surgery.

1. The confident child whose previous experiences in life have left him open to and interested in new experiences.
2. The apprehensive and insecure child whose limited previous experiences in life have been coloured by attitudes learnt from anxious adults but who is capable of being reconditioned with sympathetic management.
3. The emotionally damaged child, fortunately rare, who is suffering from overwhelming fear, perhaps as a result of previously unsympathetic or inadequate treatment, either dental or surgical, or a recent family disaster or other traumatic experience.

The way a child behaves and co-operates in the dental surgery is partly affected by his general life-style, e.g. family attitudes, friend's experience, general trait towards anxiety and so on, but it is influenced more profoundly and specifically by previous painful experiences during medical or dental treatment, and by prolonged appointments which were beyond the particular child's endurance.

Physically or mentally handicapped children will need special consideration and care based on the advice of the dental surgeon and medical specialist in each individual case.

GENERAL APPROACH

Parents should be encouraged to bring their children to the dental surgery for regular check-ups at four-monthly intervals from the age of two when any possible treatment needs are minimal and simple to carry out while introducing the child to the routines of dentistry.

Reception

The waiting room should have some materials in it that are specially designed for children, which may range from such things as small tables and chairs and large toys such as a rocking horse, to simply an assortment of comic books and papers. These familiar objects will allow a child to identify with its new surroundings more quickly. Whatever is provided should be sturdy, noise-free and inexpensive to replace. Some practices arrange to see all child patients at special sessions and then the waiting room can be specifically arranged for children. Remember that it is often the parent who has to wait there so make sure that there are some adult magazines available as well. Early morning appointments are best for young children for they are generally more co-operative when they are not tired or hungry.

185

The DSA is the first person that the child meets in the dental situation, so make sure that you know his first name readily and that you greet him with a smile, a kind but firm voice and a sympathetic manner. Make sure that his parent gives him the opportunity to visit the toilet before he goes into the surgery. Listen to anything that the parent wants to say about the child's general or dental health and never neglect to tell the dental surgeon about it, particularly any complaint about the teeth that the child has made at home. Try not to discuss possible treatment in front of the child or he may be left with half-understood details for his active imagination to work on. Do not keep children waiting very long, for their ability to co-operate starts to run out from the moment they arrive at the dental surgery whether or not they are receiving treatment. Remember that early treatment sets the pattern of attitude for life and that everyone should strive to make the visits to the dental surgery a routine, almost enjoyable, event and not an ordeal to be avoided as long as possible.

Be on the alert for communicable childhood diseases that might possibly be transmitted to other patients. One important example is the simple childhood disease of rubella (German measles) which, if transmitted to a susceptible expectant mother can severely affect the development of her unborn child.

In the dental surgery

The dental surgeon will decide if a particular parent should accompany the child into the surgery, but usually this is only necessary for very young children, or for a first consultation. The parent should be provided with a seat that does not impede the treatment area of the surgery.

Once the child is in the dental surgery the DSA should continue to maintain a general atmosphere of sympathetic support, but neither she nor the parent must distract the child's attention either verbally or by their actions, from what the dental surgeon is saying. If all three adults are talking at once, the nervous child will become confused and afraid. The team approach remains important. The chair is adjusted to suit the child and any movement or tilting of the chair announced in advance. Very few child-sized instruments are required for routine dental care and these are generally limited to small handpiece heads and miniature burs, small saliva ejector tips, small diameter cotton-wool rolls and small matrix holders.

Treatment should be carried out in an atmosphere of quiet, unhurried and deliberate progress with the minimum of wasted time and effort. Many procedures can be carried out with a minimum of simple instruments to avoid delays. Each new procedure is explained to the child in simple understandable terms and he is warned in advance of noises, tastes and unusual sensations.

Case histories and subsequent treatment planning need the presence of a parent, not only to give a satisfactory account of the child's medical and dental history, but in order that future treatment can be discussed and that parental consent to a course of treatment is obtained. If a general anaesthetic or relative analgesia will be required, the parent or guardian's written consent must be obtained. Consent to local anaesthesia, considered to be a routine treatment procedure, is implied if the parent makes an appointment for their child at the dental surgery, but if possible the parent should be informed that it is to be given. It is always advisable to consult the parent first if any extensive or irreversible treatment such as an extraction or crown preparation is necessary.

CONSERVATION TREATMENT IN THE PRIMARY TEETH

Early detection of dental caries in the primary dentition requires regular dental check-ups and at least annual bite-wing radiographs.

The dental anatomy of the primary teeth has to be taken into account during the treatment of caries and its complications in the primary dentition. The teeth are small and barrel-shaped with thin layers of enamel and dentine overlying a pulp which has long pulp horns extending into the dentine. The root canals of the molars have a complex curved structure and the root apices of all primary teeth lie in close proximity to the forming permanent successors.

Treatment of caries

Caries in the primary teeth may be treated in three ways:
1. Topical applications of fluorides have been shown to arrest the caries process in very early lesions. Stannous fluoride or acidulated fluoride phosphate solutions are applied to cleaned and dried carious surfaces.
2. Modification of the shape of the tooth. Overhanging enamel at the margins of cavities may be smoothed away with sandpaper discs and abrasive stones and the cavity 'saucerised' to remove the bulk of caries and to make it self-cleansing in an attempt to stop the carious process. This means a considerable loss of tooth structure and poor aesthetic appearance.
3. Restoration of the tooth. This is the recommended treatment. All the caries is removed and a cavity is prepared by conventional means so that the tooth may be filled and restored to function and appearance. The preparations have to be shallow to avoid pulpal exposure and are often made wider than in permanent teeth to allow sufficient bulk of material to be inserted to produce a strong restoration. Deep cavities are generally lined with a thin calcium hydroxide cement. In Class II restorations a wedged matrix must be used to prevent the production of a cervical overhanging edge. Restoration of the incisor teeth is

particularly difficult where the incisal angle has been lost. Restorative materials for the primary teeth include amalgam, zinc-free amalgam, phosphate, silico-phosphate, glass ionomer cements, composite resins and, more rarely, even gold or silver inlays. Very broken-down or potentially weak teeth can be restored by fitting a stainless steel crown form over them which has been contoured with specially designed pliers at the chairside.

Pulp therapy techniques

These can preserve a great many valuable primary teeth that would otherwise have to be extracted long before natural exfoliation should occur, because of pulpal exposure or other pathological condition.

This form of treatment can only be carried out on selected teeth after careful clinical consideration and radiographic examination. The child must be sufficiently co-operative to accept this slightly prolonged type of treatment and should have no general physical or medical contra-indication. The numerous techniques vary in detail but fall into four main categories.

Pulp capping. Direct pulp capping of the primary teeth is usually unsuccessful. It can only hope to succeed in the rarely occurring ideal conditions in which the pulp is vital, the exposure small, non-infected and surrounded by non-infected dentine. The exposure is covered with a calcium hydroxide paste, the cavity lined with cement and then filled permanently at the same sitting.

Vital pulpotomy. This is the method of choice with an exposed vital pulp in a primary tooth. Under local anaesthesia and dry, isolated and aseptic conditions the pulp chamber is opened up and its contents removed with a sterile excavator. The amputated ends of the vital pulp tissue remaining in the root canals are then covered with calcium hydroxide paste and the tooth lined and filled permanently.

Devitalising pulpotomy. If the pulp is vital, but there is evidence of infection in the pulp chamber, the tooth is first prepared as for a vital pulpotomy. Then a pledget of cotton-wool moistened with formo-cresol is placed in the cavity for two minutes to sterilise the surface. The pledget is removed and a stiff paste, made up of formo-cresol, eugenol and zinc oxide powder, is placed in the pulp chamber, and the tooth lined and filled permanently.

Root filling. Where the pulp of a primary tooth is infected and non-vital, extraction of the tooth is usually considered. However, in some cases it is still possible to carry out treatment to prolong its safe retention in the

188

mouth. The disadvantage of this method is that the dental anatomy of the primary molar does not allow thorough mechanical preparation of the root canal in the way that it can be carried out on a permanent tooth. The exposed tooth is opened up widely, the dead pulp tissue is removed to eliminate as much of the infected material as possible and a pledget of cotton-wool, soaked in disinfectant such as camphorated mono-chlorophenol, is firmly sealed into the cavity for three or four days. If all is well clinically, the tooth is then opened up again, the dressing removed, the pulp chamber filled with a resorbable antiseptic paste and the tooth restored permanently.

In every case the tooth has to be kept under careful observation both clinically and radiographically and the patient must return immediately should pain, discomfort or swelling occur in the region of the treated tooth.

TRAUMATIC INJURIES TO THE TEETH

Almost 10 per cent of children will damage their teeth in falls, contact sports, street accidents and other mishaps and most of these injuries are to the incisor region of the mouth. Predisposing factors include protruding teeth, slow reaction times to ward off the injury, poor eyesight and a general knockabout, accident-prone disposition. The injury often seems more severe to the parent and the child than it really merits and prompt and efficient treatment is greatly appreciated by them. Sometimes it is difficult to get the exact story of the accident out of a frightened child, for they tend to minimise a misdemeanor for fear of punishment. It is wise, therefore to look at the whole child first before proceeding to examine the mouth, to make sure that a more severe yet deliberately concealed injury has not taken place that will require urgent medical or hospital attention.

The clinical examination sets out to discover the extent of the injury both to the bones of the skull, face and jaws and to the soft tissues overlying them, particularly the nose and lips. The extent of the loosening or fracture of the teeth is noted and any cuts or tears in the oral mucosa and tongue. Thermal and electrical tests are carried out to determine the extent of the injury to the pulps of the teeth involved. Radiographs are always taken to check for possible injuries to the roots of the teeth and the extent of any displacement from their sockets. Larger films of the skull and jaws may be needed on occasion and sometimes special films of the lip or tongue will reveal that a part of the fractured tooth has been driven into them.

Classification of traumatic injuries to teeth
1. Fracture of the enamel.
2. Fracture involving the dentine.
3. Fracture exposing the pulp.

4. Fracture of the root.
5. Tooth displaced in the socket.

Treatment

Obviously general care of the injured child, and the arrest of any haemorrhage will take priority. Then the dental treatment may be undertaken; sometimes a tooth is so badly broken that it has to be extracted. Apart from such emergency, treatment is generally aimed at maintaining the pulp's vitality if possible (or, where this is indicated, taking steps to treat or remove it); at restoring the periodontal attachment as soon as possible after the injury and supporting the tooth until re-attachment has taken place; and, finally, restoring the tooth to function and good aesthetic appearance.

Emergency treatment. A tooth that has been completely knocked out must be returned to its socket as quickly as possible if it is to have any chance of recovery. The sharp edges of fractured enamel are smoothed down. Temporary crown forms filled with sedative cement are put over exposed dentine. Exposed pulps are either treated by capping, vital pulpotomy or pulpectomy. Teeth that have been moved in their sockets are supported using a range of splinting techniques from temporary metal foil cemented over the repositioned tooth to vacuum-formed plastic or silver cap splints made in the laboratory. Soft tissue wounds are sutured and unsaveable teeth removed. Systemic therapy such as antibiotics or anti-tetanus treatment is sometimes required for deep, possibly infected wounds.

Semi-permanent treatment. Once the initial healing has taken place, any bruising or swelling has resolved and the final condition of recovery of the pulp and periodontal structure assessed, the semi-permanent treatment can be carried out. This is based on the minimum operative interference with the young growing tissue that will give the maximum function and best aesthetic appearance.

Fractured enamel at the incisal edge can often be ground and contoured at intervals over a period of months until the fractured tooth is an acceptable shape. Loss of more extensive amounts of tooth substance requires restoration, usually with the acid etch composite technique which has now almost completely superseded the use of faced gold inlays, basket crowns and stainless steel crowns.

Acid etch technique. The enamel surface of the tooth is etched with acid, and then a composite resin used which polymerises to mechanically interlock with the roughened surface giving a microstructure bonding and increased retention. This method expands the use of composite materials for restoring tooth structure so that they may also be used in otherwise nonretentive situations, and for periodontal splinting, temporary retention of orthodontic appliances and covering or veneering malformed teeth.

1. The surface of the tooth is thoroughly cleaned and, where necessary, the fractured enamel margins bevelled with a diamond engine instrument.
2. The tooth is isolated and dried and any exposed dentine protected with a layer of calcium hydroxide cement.
3. The enamel surface is etched where necessary by applying an acid solution for 60 seconds.
4. The tooth is washed thoroughly with water and again dried, when the matt surface of the etched enamel can be seen.
5. Activated enamel bonding resin is applied to the etched surface.
6. The correct shade of composite filling material is mixed and applied over the bonding agent, controlled by a cellulose acetate crown form or matrix.
7. When set, the matrix is removed and the composite restoration finished following the manufacturer's instructions (see Chapter 8).

Splinted teeth. Where a displaced tooth has been splinted it will take several weeks before re-attachment will be firm enough to stand occlusal stress; however, the sooner the tooth can be returned to function the better. If the pulp dies during this time the tooth has to be root treated through the surface of the splint.

Where a tooth with a fractured root has been splinted no union between the fragments can occur, and success depends upon the strength of root attachment that can be achieved for the crown-supporting fragment so that the tooth can withstand normal masticatory stresses. In certain cases the root fragments can be splinted permanently by root-filling the tooth with a stainless steel pin.

Extraction. If a traumatised tooth has to be extracted the space may be retained by fitting an immediate denture with the possibility of making a bridge in later years, or the gap may be closed up by orthodontic treatment and the tooth now occupying the space ground or crowned to give a more pleasing appearance.

Permanent treatment. Permanent restoration of these injuries may not be possible until the child has reached its middle teens to allow the teeth and tissues to complete their growth and because some treatment, e.g. crowns and bridgework, is too time-consuming for a child to tolerate it.

Chapter Sixteen

ORTHODONTICS

Orthodontics is the branch of dentistry concerned primarily with the prevention or correction of irregularities in position of teeth. It includes the study of the patterns of growth and development of the teeth, jaws and face and also the function of the oro-facial soft tissues particularly in swallowing, speech and respiration.

Early diagnosis of irregularities of development of the teeth and jaws is essential if effective treatment is to be carried out in its simplest form. Although some abnormalities will not require or justify treatment, others, if neglected, may upset the quality of the child's life by undermining his future dental health or making him unhappy and self-conscious about his appearance.

Variations in teeth and jaw relationships
The teeth may vary from the normal in *number* (e.g. supernumerary or additional teeth, anodontia or the non-development of teeth); in *shape* (e.g. gemination or fusion of two teeth, peg-shaped teeth); in *size* or *position* (e.g. inclination, rotation, impaction). There may be *crowding* or *spacing* of the teeth. There may be abnormalities of the *arch shape* or the *arch relationship* between the upper and lower jaws.

Definitions
Occlusion means the relationship and contact between the upper and lower teeth upon closure of the jaws.
Normal occlusion occurs when all the teeth are present in the arches and they meet one another in a normal manner.
Malocclusion means abnormal occlusion in which teeth are not in a normal position in relation to adjacent teeth in the same jaw and/or the opposing teeth when the jaws are closed.
Pre-normal occlusion is a malocclusion where the lower teeth meet the upper teeth in front of the normal position.

192

Post-normal occlusion is where the lower teeth meet the upper teeth behind the normal position.

Overjet is the horizontal overlap of upper over lower incisors.

Overbite is the vertical overlap of upper over lower incisors.

Edge-to-edge bite occurs where there is no overlap and the incisor tips occlude.

Cross-bite occurs when one or both maxillary buccal segments (premolars and molars) are lingually displaced in occlusion.

Open bite is a condition where a space exists between the upper and lower incisor or posterior teeth when the mouth is closed.

Freeway space is the space (approximately 2mm) or clearance between the occlusal surfaces of the teeth when the mandible is in the physiological rest position.

ANGLE'S CLASSIFICATION OF MALOCCLUSION (Fig. 16/1)

Angle (1899) based his classification of dental irregularities on the antero-posterior relationship of the posterior permanent teeth in which the maxillary first permanent molar was regarded as fixed in a constant and normal position, the classification being determined by the relationship of the mandibular molar occluded to it.

CLASS I

CLASS II
div. i

CLASS II
div. ii

CLASS III

Fig. 16/1 Angle's classification of malocclusion

193

Class I

The mandibular arch is in a normal antero-posterior relationship to the maxillary arch. The mesio-buccal cusp of the maxillary first permanent molar occludes with the buccal groove of the mandibular first permanent molar.

Class II

The mandibular arch occludes too far back compared with the maxillary arch.

Division I: This occurs when the maxillary incisors are tilted forwards (proclinated).

Division 2: This occurs when the maxilliary incisors are tilted backwards (retroclinated).

Class III

The mandibular arch occludes too far forward compared with the maxillary arch.

CAUSES OF MALOCCLUSION

Positional irregularities of the teeth and the jaw relationship may be caused by general and local factors.

General factors

These can affect the development of the dental arches as a whole and include hereditary factors, the structure of the facial skeleton (skeletal pattern), the form and activity of the facial soft tissues and the size and shape of the teeth. Malformation may include hare lip and cleft palate. There may be birth injuries, malnutrition, disease or injury.

Local factors

These are the factors which affect the development of the dental arches only at specific points. For example, bottle feeding, missing teeth, supernumerary teeth, premature loss or prolonged retention of the primary teeth, impaction, loss of permanent teeth, lip and tongue behaviour, thumb or finger sucking and local disease (e.g. tumours) or injury, may all cause malocclusion.

Diagnosis. Each case requires very full examination because orthodontic problems are often caused by a very complex sequence of events.

A thorough case history is required with special emphasis upon hereditary and congenital factors and also any habits such as thumb-sucking that will affect the shape of the jaws.

The child is examined in the usual way, but with particular attention to the soft tissues of the face and oral cavity (e.g. lips and tongue shape and behaviour, swallowing patterns) and the occlusion.

The special examination requires impressions for study models and radiographs. In addition to intra-oral films, left and right lateral oblique or orthopantomogram, and occlusal films are generally required to assess the size, root shape and position of unerupted teeth. Specialist orthodontists may also require a standard position lateral skull radiograph for *cephalometric analysis* of the skeletal pattern to be made by measuring certain planes, lines and angles between standard reference points on the skull.

When all this information is available, the orthodontist can complete his diagnosis and make a treatment plan. This must be discussed in detail with the child and his parents so that their full co-operation and consent is assured before long-term treatment is started.

Indications for treatment

Orthodontic treatment is indicated in cases where the present and future function, appearance and health of the orofacial structure is affected:
1. When the abnormality interferes with masticatory function or speech.
2. Where the aesthetic appearance is poor.
3. Where the malposition or malocclusion predisposes towards caries, periodontal disease or temporomandibular joint disorders.
4. Where the abnormality may increase the risk of root resorption, tooth impaction or accidental trauma to the teeth.
5. Where good co-operation and interest from the patient and his parents are to be expected.

METHODS OF TREATMENT

Basically, orthodontic treatment falls into the following four categories.

Elimination of causative habits

This can be done by reasoning with the older child and perhaps constructing a simple appliance to help him to break the habit. Habits such as thumb-sucking in the mixed dentition period have a deep psychological basis and treatment should be aimed at the cause rather than the outward habit itself.

195

Operative treatment

(a) By extracting teeth to relieve crowding or by the extraction of retained deciduous teeth.

(b) By operating on the soft tissues (e.g. fraenectomy) or bone (e.g. altering the contour of the mandible).

(c) By selective grinding. Removal of cusps can sometimes allow an erupting tooth to move into the correct place.

Appliances

The bone supporting the teeth is a living substance that reacts to the forces placed upon it by muscular and other stresses. Teeth and groups of teeth can be moved into new positions by the use of continual pressure sufficient to cause the bone to be remodelled. These changes can be achieved more rapidly in growing children and young people. The pressure upon the teeth must not exceed certain limits or the vitality of the tooth and the adjacent periodontal membrane may be affected. In appliance therapy the pressure must be applied accurately and be under complete control while based on a firm anchorage. This *anchorage* may be gained by the use of a removable plate or a fixed metal appliance attached to groups of teeth, or from an extra-oral anchorage such as a webbing cap to which wires from the mouth can be attached.

Active appliances exert pressure on the teeth to be moved and must be kept under frequent revision by the dental surgeon. The pressure may be continuous, as with metal springs or elastic bands, or it may be intermittent, as when small screws systems are incorporated into the appliance and turned at intervals to 'wedge' the tooth or group of teeth into position.

Passive appliances do not exert a pressure and are used to retain teeth in a desired position at certain stages of treatment.

Functional appliances train muscles or else use muscle pressure to mould bone.

Fixed appliances. Stainless steel tape is formed into bands contoured to fit individual teeth. Arch wires, brackets, springs and so on, are attached to the steel bands by welding and soldering on a model and finally the whole assembly is cemented on to the teeth. (In some cases, since the advent of the polycarboxylate cements, plastic brackets are cemented directly on to the teeth and the necessary wires attached in the mouth.) These appliances can exert a continual effect upon the teeth and thus, although they have a poor appearance and are hard to keep clean, the desired effect is quickly obtained. (An orthodontic 'spot-welder' is an electrical apparatus used to weld thin stainless wires or tapes during construction of these appliances in the dental surgery or laboratory.)

Removable appliances. These are usually constructed of acrylic with stainless steel arch wires, clasps and springs. Being removable they allow normal oral hygiene procedures and can be taken out for adjustment at intervals. In certain cases they need to be worn only at night. A removable appliance can easily be lost, damaged or forgotten by the patient.

The *Norwegian plate* (Andresen appliance or Monobloc) is constructed to act as a functional appliance. It uses muscular power to re-position teeth as it directs their movement and eruption. The single acrylic plate is fitted to both arches and draws the mandible into the desired position as well as producing and directing forces upon individual and groups of teeth.

The *Frankel appliance* consists of a series of acrylic flanges joined by a stainless steel wire framework. Like the Andresen, this appliance contacts both upper and lower teeth at the same time and is generally worn only at night.

(A wide range of orthodontic pliers is available for use in the construction, contouring and adjustment of the metal wires and tapes of various dimensions that are used in most appliances.)

Chapter Seventeen

PREVENTIVE DENTISTRY

Preventive dentistry is the science and practice of measures to prevent the onset of diseases of the teeth and neighbouring soft tissues.

The commonest dental diseases are dental caries and the periodontal diseases and, to a very great extent, they can be prevented, halted or their effects minimised if appropriate action is taken early enough.

By tradition the dental surgeon and his patient have been almost completely preoccupied by the practical problems of treating the effects of already established dental disease. One course of treatment inevitably followed the next. It is only in recent years that real progress has been made in changing their attitudes so that an effort is also made to preserve an existing healthy state by taking definite action.

Most people sitting in the dental chair are easily convinced of the advantages of having a healthy and comfortable mouth, but they may need to be repeatedly reminded about it during trouble-free periods if they are to remain sufficiently motivated to carry out the necessary regular long-term effort to gain and maintain this condition.

Formation of sound teeth

The potential size and structure of the teeth is inherited from the parents, but the formation and calcification, and thus the resistance to caries, can be affected by external influences of diet and general disease.

The cells of the baby's future teeth germs start to proliferate as early as the sixth week of pregnancy and mineralisation of the primary teeth commences at about the fourth month. At birth a considerable part of the primary teeth crowns are already completed. The permanent teeth start to mineralise at birth and by seven to eight years the crowns of all but the third molars are completely calcified although the root formation continues well into adolescence.

It is important from the dental point of view that both the expectant mother and the growing child have an adequate, balanced diet containing ample proteins, fats, minerals (especially calcium) and vitamins A, C and D if strong tooth formation is to occur. The caries-resisting effects of the trace element fluorine should be considered in this context.

General physical disturbances such as gastro-enteritis, measles, jaundice and the administration of some drugs such as the tetracyclines, as well as local infections in a baby's mouth can upset the processes of tooth formation and mineralisation so that teeth erupt with ill-formed (hypoplastic) or stained enamel. Thus some of these conditions can leave the teeth very vulnerable to caries attack.

Protection of sound dental tissues

The first stage in the process of dental caries occurs when strongly adherent *dental plaque* (a film of bacteria, mucin from saliva, desquamated cells and food debris) is allowed to form on the surfaces of the erupted teeth. The presence of plaque also indicates a poor standard of oral hygiene that is commonly a precursor of gingivitis and periodontal disease. Subsequently, during and after the mastication of carbohydrates, the organisms produce a high acid concentration and the associated enamel begins to break down.

Much of practical preventive dentistry is aimed at removing or reducing dental plaque and minimising the exposure of the teeth to refined carbohydrates.

Diet control. All sugary food and drink containing fermentable carbohydrates represent a danger to the teeth, not related to the quantity of sugary material consumed as much as the frequency and duration of time that the teeth are exposed to it.

Bottle-fed babies should be weaned gradually to drinking from a cup by the time they are one year old, otherwise the sweetened milk, vitamin syrups and fruit juices that trickle slowly over the newly erupted primary teeth will result in rampant caries within a few months. This will particularly affect the teeth of the older child who is 'got off to sleep' with a bottle in the pram or cot, or who is comforted and quietened during the day with a dummy or pacifier dipped in jam or syrup, or has a longer-acting reservoir pacifier containing sugary solutions. The same danger arises with sugary medicines, especially when they are given at night. Parents should be made aware of these dangers to an infant's teeth.

Ideally, everyone should eat ample well-balanced meals at regular intervals and thus not require the between-meals snacks that can be so damaging to the teeth. If possible a meal should be finished off with a savoury food to counteract the sugar's acid-forming effects in the plaque. The child who has an unlimited quantity of sweets and spends much of his waking day with one slowly dissolving in his mouth, or the man who is trying to give up smoking and seeks an alternative oral pacification of his psychological stresses by an endless series of peppermints are both running a high risk of rampant caries.

It is hard to deprive children of sweets altogether, particularly in the face of constant persuasive advertising techniques to sell them. An alternative to prohibition has been suggested; the child may have one sweet-eating orgy a week, say Saturday afternoon, when he may eat as many sweets as he wishes for the limited period and then follow this somewhat dentally hazardous escapade by very thorough and vigorous oral hygiene. At all other times, any craving between meals should be satisfied with cheese, fruit, nuts, potato crisps and other attractive food products that are not caries-promoting.

The importance of diet control can be emphasised by arranging for the patient or the child's parent to keep a written record of all food and drink consumed over the period of a week, noting times and quantities. Subsequent discussion about this record with the dental surgeon, as they check to identify sugary foods and recommend acceptable non-sugary alternatives, will do much to bring the whole matter to the level of conscious thought and choice in future.

Oral hygiene. Everyone must be made conscious of the need to carry out regular oral hygiene: a clean mouth feels fresh and comfortable, improves the appearance and is socially pleasant. Simple daily care removes stains, polishes the surface and margins of restorations and does much to maintain a good periodontal condition and prevent halitosis (bad breath). There are, however, limitations to the extent to which this method can reduce the onset of caries attack. Although 'a clean tooth never decays' and there is ample evidence that tooth brushing can prevent or even arrest white-spot caries on accessible surfaces, the structure of the teeth at the contact points, pits and fissures is such that no known method of oral hygiene can make a perfect job of removing all the dental plaque. Oral hygiene is of use in preventing dental caries only if it is practised at the same time as a method of diet control to minimise the activity of the undisturbed plaque in inaccessible situations.

Toothbrushing should be carried out regularly at least after breakfast and last thing at night. Generally, the toothbrush should have a short head, a flat bristle surface and a firm non-bending handle. The bristles should be of medium hard animal bristle or nylon (unless another hardness is recommended by the dental surgeon) and must be allowed to dry out completely after each period of use or they will become softened and unsuitable for the task.

Toothpastes contain abrasive and detergent agents that assist the cleaning effect of the brush.

Toothbrushing techniques have to be adapted to suit each individual's mouth. The methods of brushing an intact arch will differ from those where several teeth have been lost or for a child in the mixed dentition stage. Parents must brush their children's teeth themselves, or finish it off, or supervise the procedure depending on the child's age, at least once a day.

Brushing back and forth in a mesio-distal direction is bad both for the gingivae and the damaging effect it will have on the thin enamel that covers the necks of the teeth. Many different techniques for brushing the teeth have been recommended. One method recommended for general use is the circular scrub where the bristles are placed against a segment of teeth with the bristles at an angle of 45° to the tooth surface and the tips of the bristles carried into the spaces between the teeth and the gums; the brush head is then moved in a circular path to clean that segment before moving to the next. Another method is to brush the teeth the way they grow, from the gingival margin to the tip of the tooth, using sweeping strokes. This action must be repeated both on the buccal and labial surfaces and on the lingual and palatal surfaces taking great care not to miss an area. After this the biting surfaces should be brushed thoroughly, and finally the loosened particles of food debris should be rinsed out of the mouth with plenty of water. Thorough toothbrushing will be easier if it is carried out while looking in a mirror to check the results visually. A most effective aid to ensure good oral hygiene is the *disclosing solution* or tablet which is introduced into the mouth before brushing commences and colours all food debris and plaque bright red. The teeth are then to be brushed by an approved method until all the stained material has been removed.

Single-tufted, or interspace toothbrushes can be used for stimulating small areas of gingivae between particular teeth or for cleaning otherwise inaccessible areas of the mouth, such as around fixed bridgework.

Mains and battery-powered electric toothbrushes can be used to clean the teeth very thoroughly and quickly with the minimum of effort and require little manual dexterity to manipulate them into various places in the mouth.

Interdental cleaning. The spaces between the teeth usually cannot be reached by the bristles of a conventional toothbrush. Trapped food particles may be cleaned from the interdental space by sliding a length of waxed *dental floss* carefully between the teeth and then moving it gently up and down, pressing it first against one tooth and then the other. This method is particularly useful for dislodging fragments of fibrous food such as meat or apple skin that have become wedged between the teeth.

Another method involves the use of specially shaped *wood points*. These are made of firm or soft wood and the patient must be advised which is suitable for his personal use. They are only to be used where the interdental papillae do not fill the interdental space in a healthy mouth. The wood point is passed gently between the teeth, low down at gingival level and moved back and forth to dislodge food debris and at the same time massage the interdental papilla to stimulate and harden the otherwise inaccessible epithelial surface.

Water can be used in an attempt to wash bulky food debris from between the teeth but cannot, of course, remove dental plaque. A small quantity is taken into the mouth, forced repeatedly between the tongue and the cheek via the interdental spaces and then swallowed or spat out. *Oral irrigation* machines are available that produce a strong, pulsating jet of water or mouthwash through a fine nozzle that can be directed against the surface of the teeth and through the interdental space with considerable cleansing effect.

Regular dental inspections. Everyone should have a thorough dental examination at regular intervals. As a general rule adults should be examined every six months and expectant mothers and children, who are potentially more caries prone, should be dentally examined every four months. Once a patient's course of treatment is completed and he has been brought to a state of dental health, his name should be placed on a recall list or at least he should be advised to seek a further inspection after the recommended interval. These regular dental check-ups are a sound principle of preventive dentistry for they mean that any carious lesions, periodontal disorders, etc, are discovered early before they can deteriorate. This will ensure that any treatment needed is minimal and simple to carry out and thus visits to the dental surgery remain pleasant, acceptable and unlikely to cause fear and apprehension.

Fluorides. It has been discovered that if a minute trace of the element fluorine is available to the child's body during the period that the teeth are formed and mineralised, then the enamel formed is stronger and more resistant to dental caries. In some parts of the world fluorides are present naturally in the drinking water and it has been shown that people born and bred there have a much lower caries rate than average. Excessive amounts of fluoride, on the other hand, can upset the normal formation of the enamel with resultant mottling of the teeth. It is known that one part per million of fluoride in the drinking water is the best for partial control of dental caries. It is suggested that some 55 to 60 per cent reduction is achieved in this way. Where water supplies have not been fluoridated, tablets containing fluoride can be taken every day during the period of tooth formation with possibly a 50 per cent reduction of caries. Topical application of fluoride to erupted teeth in the form of freshly made up solutions or in a gel or lacquer can give a 20 to 30 per cent reduction, while the daily use of a toothpaste containing fluorides (0.2% sodium fluoride) or rinsing the mouth with a very dilute solution can give a caries reduction of 20 to 30 per cent. Sometimes a combination of internal and topical use of fluoride can be suggested as a doubly effective method of gaining this benefit.

Fissure sealants. Plastic materials have been developed which may be used to seal pits and fissures of non-carious teeth for long periods and thus eliminate potential danger spots where plaque can collect undisturbed.

1. The teeth to be treated are cleaned with an oil-free, non-fluoride polishing paste and washed thoroughly.
2. A quadrant of teeth is isolated with cotton-wool rolls and the teeth thoroughly dried with the air syringe.
3. The etching solution is applied to the surfaces with a cotton-wool pledget for 60 seconds.
4. The teeth are washed thoroughly (carefully avoiding saliva contamination), the tooth dried with air, and new cotton-wool rolls placed in position. The etched surfaces will appear to be whitened and frosty.
5. The selected resin is prepared according to the manufacturer's instructions and applied to the tooth fissures. (Some resins are clear and others are tinted in contrast to the enamel.)
6. After about two minutes the resin has set, and is checked for coverage, retention and occlusion with the opposing teeth before the patient is dismissed.

Once polymerised, the excess resin wears away leaving the fissures sealed. Every sealed surface should be re-examined at six-monthly intervals and re-sealed if necessary.

DENTAL HEALTH EDUCATION

The simple basic facts about methods of preventing dental disease must continually be made available to all levels of the public. Adults have to be made aware of them both for themselves and in their capacity as parents and examples to young people. Mothers and expectant mothers have a particularly important role in this respect.

All people working in health and education services, e.g. medical practitioners, welfare workers, nurses and schoolteachers, should be kept up to date with the latest facts about dental health matters so that they can pass on the information, at appropriate times, during their contact with the public.

Every member of the dental team has an individual duty to communicate this information with the direct supervision and permission of the dental surgeon, with almost missionary zeal. The basic facts are very simple. The real problem is how to motivate people to take notice and act upon the knowledge. No one in the dental team must neglect an opportunity to teach people, either as individuals or in groups of children or adults, about the importance of having a healthy mouth and the methods of gaining and maintaining it. A great deal of attractive teaching aids and materials in the form of pamphlets and books, posters, film strips, tape-slides and lecture notes, teaching models, sound movie films and so on, are readily available from the professional organisations (e.g. the General Dental Council, Health Education Council and so on). With such inspiring and motivating material to hand, no one need hesitate about their ability to pass on the message of dental health.

Other aspects of preventive dentistry. Preventive dentistry is not solely concerned with the problems of dental caries and the periodontal diseases. This attitude of prediction of events and the institution of corrective measures to achieve and maintain a healthy situation must also be brought to all other aspects of dentistry. For example, in children's dentistry irregularities of growth must be detected and forecast early so that simple corrective measures can be started and thus prevent more serious problems later on. The increasing use of mouthguards in contact sports has emphasised the value of these plastic devices in the avoidance of fractured or dislocated teeth. In prosthetics, the patient fitted with satisfactory full dentures is encouraged to return to have them checked at least every two years so that changes in the bite or damage to the oral mucosa due to loss of fit can be prevented. In the surgery, care with x-ray radiation, the reduction of possible mercury fumes, the precautions to avoid transference of infection, and so on, are all preventive measures in themselves.

Chapter Eighteen

HAZARDS AND EMERGENCIES IN THE DENTAL SURGERY

When a patient comes into the dental surgery the full responsibility for his safety and well-being is in the hands of the dental surgeon and his staff. Potential hazards, both in the environment and in treatment, must be anticipated and where possible eliminated. It is better to foresee and avoid emergencies than to have to deal with them.

THE HEALTH AND SAFETY AT WORK etc ACT 1974

This act emphasises the legal responsibility borne by employers and staff to reduce the likelihood of accidental injury or health risks at their place of work to themselves, or members of the general public (e.g. patients), in relation to work activities. This legislation introduces penalties for failing to maintain safe standards; although Codes of Practice are being drawn up by the Health and Safety Commission, everyone should be aware of the need to review current practices in the light of these legal requirements. It is quite impossible to list every potential hazard, but it is stressed that it is the personal responsibility of every member of the dental team to protect himself and others.

Any accident or defect in equipment, supplies, fixtures and fittings must be reported immediately to the head of the team, and steps taken at once to prevent a recurrence of the incident. All accidents to patients or staff must be recorded in the accident book, and should include date, time and names of staff present; to whom reported and action taken. Such records have to be kept for a minimum period of seven years.

For specific risks see Chapter 7 – radiological hazards; Chapter 8 – mercury contamination; and Chapter 12 – anaesthetic hazards.

GENERAL HAZARDS

The following cannot be comprehensive, but the examples given will show the basic preventive attitude that must be adopted by the dental team.

Furniture and fittings
Are there any unfastened linoleum or carpet edges, polished or uneven floor surfaces, loose mats or electrical cables which may cause the patient to trip, slip and fall? Are the stairs adequately lit? Are there any projecting corners of desks, shelves or cabinets that the unwary patient might knock himself against?

In all respects every member of the dental team has a responsibility and obligation to be alert to discover and take adequate steps to deal with any hazards that may put their own or other people's health and safety at risk.

Patient
Is there anything about him that will require special care and consideration? This may perhaps be a physical limitation: blindness, poor eyesight, deafness, unsteadiness on the feet or a medical condition. It may be emotional or mental: instability leading to poor co-operation during treatment or a tendency to make sudden, uncontrolled movements. All visitors to the surgery must be protected as well as the patient, e.g. a child should not be left unattended or allowed to run about the surgery while another member of the family is being treated.

Dental equipment
This must be maintained in a reliable working order so that there is no likelihood of it breaking down during treatment with resultant danger to the patient.
Electricity must be treated with respect and a constant watch kept on electric cables, wiring and plugs to avoid the possibility of electric shocks due to worn wiring or inadequately earthed equipment.
Heat is a constant hazard in the surgery. The patient must sometimes be warned about, and always protected from, gas flames, sterilisers and autoclaves. Instruments should never be 'flamed' with burning alcohol. If alcohol or other inflammable liquids are used at the chairside they should be dispensed in small quantities in a container that is kept well away from any naked flame. *Never* put stock bottles of these liquids on the bracket table.
X-ray apparatus must be used and maintained with adequate precautions (see Chapter 7).

Instruments and materials. Very rarely an instrument such as a bur or a reamer may break while being used in the patient's mouth. This danger can be minimised if care is taken to avoid weakening such instruments during sterilisation and general handling and to replace them frequently with new ones. When a breakage occurs, all the fragments must be traced and recovered, sometimes a time-consuming and worrying matter.

The patient must be protected against the common accident of dropping instruments or materials on to him. His clothes must be covered with adequate bibs and towels for the particular operation undertaken and instruments, drugs and materials should not be passed to the dental surgeon over the patient's face. Where the patient is lying flat his eyes should be protected with goggles.

All instruments must be properly sterilised to avoid the hazard of cross-infection. All drugs must be properly and clearly labelled to prevent mistakes in their use.

Consent to treatment

This must be obtained from the patient or, in the case of a minor under the age of sixteen, from his parent or responsible guardian. This consent must be in writing when a general anaesthetic is to be used. The DSA should be present in the surgery at all times during dental treatment as a witness and chaperone.

TREATMENT HAZARDS

Most hazards will be avoided when an adequate and thorough case history has been taken at the start of a course of treatment so that the patient's general health and medical condition are known. It is particularly important to know if the patient is receiving medical treatment and drugs for any reason, and further, up-to-date information must be sought from the patient each time an anaesthetic or other drug is given. Before a general anaesthetic is given always check that the patient has followed the instruction about not eating or drinking for the previous four hours.

The prevention of local complications during treatment is entirely the dental surgeon's responsibility, but the DSA must be aware of the potential hazards such as slips and cuts with sharp instruments and damage to anaesthetised parts. The patient must always be protected from the danger of swallowing or inhaling small instruments, by using, for example, rubber dam or by anchoring the instrument with a length of dental floss.

During treatment or in the immediate postoperative period the patient may suffer haemorrhage, collapse or loss of consciousness and the treatment for these emergencies is described on page 211.

Postoperative care

As soon as treatment is completed everything must be done to ensure that nothing untoward occurs during the postoperative recovery period. Patients will need time to recover themselves before being allowed to leave. Those who have had a sedative drug, an anaesthetic or prolonged treatment, may have to spend time in the recovery room and may not be fit to go home unless accompanied by a responsible adult. Patients under the influence of drugs must not be allowed to drive themselves home by car or take part in any potentially hazardous activity such as finding their own way home by public transport.

Any postoperative instructions about what to do in the event of pain, haemorrhage or infection together with the follow-up appointment should be given to the patient in writing so that he may study them later.

The DSA must confirm that all bleeding has ceased before allowing the patient to leave after an extraction.

CONDITIONS REQUIRING SPECIAL PRECAUTIONS

Anaphylactic shock

Drug sensitivity reactions can vary from mild skin rashes to severe anaphylactic shock where the patient who has been sensitised by a previous dose of a drug suffers a serious reaction to a second dose of the same drug. He feels weak and nauseated, rapidly becomes pale and loses consciousness; the sudden fall in blood pressure causes a weak pulse. He may also suffer convulsions, total collapse and even death unless immediate treatment is given.

The patient must be laid flat and the legs elevated to restore the blood pressure. Adrenaline injection (1:1000) 0.5ml is injected intramuscularly and oxygen given. An injection containing 100mg of hydrocortisone sodium succinate should be given intramuscularly. (*Note*: The DSA is *not* qualified to give an injection to a patient.)

Penicillin sensitivity is one potential cause of this wide range of reactions.

Angina

This severe pain behind the sternum is caused by a spasm of the arteries serving the heart muscle, and may be brought on by over-activity or stress. It usually lasts only a few minutes and can be relieved by the patient sucking a glyceryl trinitrate tablet. Patients suffering from angina should only be treated after consultation with their doctor.

Anticoagulants

Patients who have suffered disorders causing thrombosis (blood clots in the blood vessels) are given anticoagulant drugs to prevent further clot formation or embolus (clot fragments escaping into the general circulation). For example, a patient who has had a coronary thrombosis (heart attack) will be treated in this way. Any dental treatment, such as extractions, for such a patient will probably result in prolonged and dangerous bleeding that will require admission to hospital. This can be avoided by obtaining an adequate drug history *before* commencing treatment, and these patients usually carry a card explaining their drug regimen. Extractions can only be carried out safely after a period in which the anticoagulant drug dose is adjusted under a doctor's supervision, and the clotting time has returned to acceptable limits.

Antidepressants

A large number of patients suffering a severe and prolonged mental depression are given drugs that can improve their mood: these may be monoamine oxidase inhibitors (MAOI) or polycyclic antidepressants.

MAOI drugs may cause raised blood pressure and headaches and, rarely, brain haemorrhage, if they are taken in conjunction with certain foods, e.g. cheese, beans, Marmite, or certain drugs (e.g. some analgesics). They must be advised *not* to take these items.

Polycyclic drugs cause problems by potentiating the effects of other drugs such as adrenaline, and these patients should only have local anaesthetics which do not contain adrenaline. Children who suffer from enuresis (bed-wetting) are sometimes given these polycyclic drugs.

Cardiac infarction (coronary thrombosis)

This occurs when a blood clot or thrombus blocks one of the main end-arteries serving the muscle of the heart. There is a sudden onset of prolonged severe pain behind the sternum, perhaps radiating to the left arm and neck. The patient looks grey-faced and shocked. An ambulance should be called for immediately. The patient should remain undisturbed, lying down where possible and kept warm. Oxygen may be given. Morphine for the pain and intensive care in hospital are urgently required.

Corticosteroids

A number of medical conditions such as rheumatoid arthritis, skin and eye diseases are treated with steroid hormones. These drugs, taken over long periods, can leave the patient liable to collapse as a result of stress unless the steroid hormone dosage has been specially adjusted before a dental operation. Such patients usually carry a special medical card which should be shown to the dental surgeon. If a patient collapses in the dental surgery due to this problem he should be admitted to hospital. Emergency treatment, after consultation with a doctor, involves the administration of hydrocortisone sodium succinate. Steroid hormones lead to delay in wound healing.

Diabetes

Diabetic patients have difficulty in controlling their blood sugar levels due to a hormone (insulin) deficiency. If these levels are not adequately balanced by special diet precautions and/or the use of insulin, patients may suffer hypoglycemia (a lack of blood sugar), feel weak and hungry, become anxious and sweating, and may lose consciousness. Special precautions must be taken to maintain blood sugar levels during certain dental treatments, e.g. general anaesthesia and multiple extractions, and also in the presence of dental infections. These patients are usually treated only after consultation with their doctor.

Epilepsy

There is usually a history of previous epileptic attacks. The patient may experience an aura that warns him of an impending attack and then fall unconscious usually with convulsions. Treatment is directed towards protecting the patient from injuring himself in falling and also protecting the tongue from being bitten, until he recovers consciousness. Epilepsy may be controlled by the patient taking anti-epileptic drugs over long periods: gingival hypoplasia is a side-effect of *phenytoin*.

Heart lesions

Patients with heart lesions (e.g. heart murmurs, damaged heart valves or a history of rheumatic fever) require antibiotic cover during dental surgical treatment to prevent possible complications due to stray organisms released into the bloodstream. The precise regimen is usually advised by the patient's doctor, but penicillin or one of its derivatives (in penicillin-sensitive patients, erythromycin) is given orally to the patient about an hour before the operation, and continued over the next 24 hours. Patients who have prosthetic heart valves also require this kind of prophylaxis.

Patients who have had cardiac pacemakers fitted require special care because, very rarely, the pacemaker's action may be affected by certain electrical or ultrasonic instruments in the dental surgery.

Pregnancy

The normal expectant mother requires special consideration. Her treatment is best undertaken during the middle three months of her pregnancy and she must not be kept in the dental chair for long periods. Her comfortable positioning is important and oxygen should be available in the surgery should she faint to prevent danger to the baby. The taking of radiographs must be kept to a minimum because x-rays can affect the fetus adversely. The expectant mother should only be given drugs for good reasons, because they can pass through the placenta and affect the fetus or later pass into the mother's milk and affect the infant.

Sickle-cell anaemia

This is an inherited disease which is confined almost entirely to the negro races. Abnormal haemoglobin in the red cells causes them to assume a sickle shape at low oxygen tensions with increased blood viscosity and possible capillary thrombosis; such changes may cause risk to life. Any patients who may be thought to fall into this group should have had a blood test to ascertain whether they have the condition before they are given a general anaesthetic.

EMERGENCIES

HAEMORRHAGE

This is the escape of blood from the blood vessels, and may be *primary* when it occurs at the time of the injury, or during surgery, due to the cutting of blood vessels; *reactionary* when it occurs after the blood pressure, reduced during a period of shock after an injury, rises again; or *secondary* when it occurs as a result of infection of the wound and breakdown of the vessels before permanent repair has taken place, usually seven to ten days later. The bleeding may be *arterial*, from a severed artery, when the blood is bright red and spurts in pulsating jets; *venous*, from a cut vein, when the blood is dark red or purple and flows continuously; or *capillary*, from the minute peripheral vessels, when the blood is red and oozes steadily but is not copious. The average healthy male can lose 570–850ml (1–1½ pints) and only feel weak, whereas a sick or elderly person or a child may suffer considerably from the loss of a much smaller amount.

Temporary arrest of haemorrhage. This takes place by the self-sealing coagulation of blood in the opening of the cut vessels and in arteries this is aided by the contraction of the muscular walls of the severed vessel. In certain diseases, e.g. haemophilia, jaundice, the coagulation mechanism of the blood is impaired.

When a lot of blood is lost suddenly, the general blood pressure falls and the remaining blood coagulates more readily. The dangers of the reduction of blood volume are counteracted by a general vasoconstriction of the peripheral blood vessels of the body to maintain supplies to the vital heart-lung-brain circulation.

Permanent arrest of haemorrhage. This takes place when the blood clot or thrombus is replaced by organised fibrous tissue during the general healing of the injured part.

211

Treatment
The *local treatment* of bleeding depends upon the type of haemorrhage and the position and extent of the injury.

Arterial haemorrhage. The immediate first-aid treatment of this dangerous condition is to apply firm finger or thumb, *digital*, pressure to the bleeding point, preferably protecting the wound from infection by a sterile gauze swab. If this fails the main artery to the injured part must be compressed against an underlying bone if possible. (Arterial haemorrhage from the tongue may be controlled by pulling the tongue forward and compressing the lingual arteries against the mandible.) Subsequent deliberate surgical treatment may involve suturing the wound or even gripping the bleeding vessel with artery forceps and then tying off the open end with a ligature.

Venous haemorrhage. This is controlled by direct digital or other pressure to the bleeding point for about five minutes.

Capillary haemorrhage. This is not usually severe and stops spontaneously in most cases.

Haemorrhage immediately following dental extraction can usually be controlled by not allowing the patient to rinse the mouth with water and getting him to bite on a firm, sterile pack for a few minutes so that the socket is filled with undisturbed blood clot. Where the bleeding persists it may be controlled by suturing the wound or by the use of haemostatic (coagulation producing) drugs or resorbable haemostatic packs that can be introduced into the socket. When a vasoconstricting local anaesthetic has been used to infiltrate a region before surgery, reactionary haemorrhage can occur when the effect wears off. Other common causes of post-extraction bleeding include excessive mouth washing, very hot food and drink, alcohol and excessive bodily activity during the recovery period.

First-aid treatment of post-extraction bleeding
The patient should be reassured, a cold mouth wash may be given to help remove excessive blood clots from other regions of the mouth, the bleeding point located and the patient given a sterile pack to bite on while the dental surgeon is called.

FAINTING (syncope)

This is the commonest general complication to occur in the dental surgery. However, the first signs and symptoms of this condition are similar to those of the more serious emergencies of respiratory failure, circulatory collapse and heart failure and the diagnosis of fainting may only be confirmed when the patient begins to respond to simple first-aid treatment.

Fainting may be caused by an unpleasant sensation such as severe pain or emotional stimulation such as fear or surprise, and may be more likely to occur in a hot, airless atmosphere or as a result of severe haemorrhage. It is due to the over-reaction of the vasomotor centres in the brain, which control the blood pressure, so that blood is diverted to the peripheral circulation and the brain is deprived of blood. The signs and symptoms are those of lack of oxygen to the brain. The patient feels distressed, weak, dizzy and nauseated. The skin becomes pale, sweaty and cold. The pulse rate is rapid and thin and the patient either shows signs of brain stimulation or depression. The pallor and sweating increase and the patient loses consciousness. The blood pressure falls and the pulse slows. The continued reduction of oxygen to the brain may cause involuntary muscle-twitching or even convulsions.

Treatment
1. At the first sign of fainting the patient should be placed in a horizontal position. If he is in a dental chair this may be tilted so that the head and heart are at a lower level than the legs. In this way the blood pressure to the brain is immediately raised by gravity.
2. Tight clothing around the neck should be loosened and a reflex respiratory stimulant such as ammonia smelling salts administered at intervals.
3. If consciousness is lost, administer oxygen by mask until the patient's colour returns to normal.
4. If recovery does not occur within a few minutes a more serious condition must be suspected and medical aid should be called. The patient's pulse and respiration rate should be kept under constant observation.

RESPIRATORY FAILURE

All respiration may stop and the patient will rapidly become *cyanosed* with blue lips and oral mucosa as the heart continues to circulate inadequately oxygenated blood through the body.

Treatment
1. Place the patient flat on his back on a firm surface, preferably the floor, checking his colour, chest movements and the carotid pulse.
2. Put the patient's head well back, drawing the jaw forward and supporting it. This brings the tongue forward, clear of the airway and may be all that is required to start the patient breathing again. Loosen any tight clothing at the patient's neck.

3. Clear the air passages of nose, mouth and throat. If the patient has loose dentures remove them, if not leave them in place as they help to give the mouth a better shape making artificial respiration easier.
4. **Mouth to mouth respiratory resuscitation** (Fig. 18/1). Inspire fully, place your mouth over the patient's mouth, pinch his nostrils closed with your fingers. Blow forcibly into his lungs, and watch the patient's chest expand each time – it should rise as the air enters the lungs.

Fig. 18/1 Mouth to mouth resuscitation: A. Inspiration; B. Expiration

5. **Mouth to nose respiratory resuscitation.** Inspire fully, place your mouth over the patient's nose, hold his jaw forward but close his mouth. Blow forcibly into the patient's lungs, and watch the patient's chest expand each time – it should rise as the air enters the lungs.
6. With either of these methods, mouth-to-mouth, or mouth-to-nose, raise your body and breathe in again while the patient expires passively.
7. Inspire deeply and repeat the sequence, giving the first four inflations as quickly as you can, and then at 12 to 20 times a minute; continue until the patient starts to breathe again, or help arrives.

If the chest does not expand after applying artificial respiration as described, it must be assumed that there is a blockage in the airway, and the oropharynx should be checked by sweeping it clear with a finger. If the blockage persists, other methods of dislodging it should be tried rapidly: (a) roll the patient on his side (a child may be inverted over the forearm) and deliver several firm blows with the heel of the hand to the spine between the shoulder blades or (b) use the *Heimlich manoeuvre* as follows: roll the patient onto his stomach (prone), straddle the lower torso, clasp both hands beneath the patient to form a fist in the mid-line and mid-way between the ribs and the navel and, in a sudden, rapid movement upward cause a rise in the pressure in the lungs that should expel any foreign body; resume artificial respiration.

Persistent blockage requires tracheostomy (where the surgeon makes an incision into the trachea to provide an accessory airway).

Note: Special airways, e.g. Brook airway, are made to conduct air from the operator to the patient without actual physical contact between the two. They are not essential and no time must be lost in looking for one in an emergency. Oxygen should be available and the dental surgeon may wish to administer a respiratory stimulant to the patient by injection.

CARDIAC ARREST

The signs of cardiac failure and circulatory collapse may swiftly follow the loss of consciousness and respiratory failure. No pulse will be felt at the wrist or in the neck, the patient's condition will be deteriorating and he will become cold and grey with the pupils of his eyes dilated. No heart sound will be heard or heart beat felt in the chest.

Cardiac arrest need not be fatal if oxygenated blood can be pumped to the brain within three minutes, after which time permanent brain damage will occur.

Treatment

Note: External cardiac compression should not be carried out unless you are sure that the heart has stopped beating.

1. Note the time and call for help.
2. Place the patient flat on his back on a firm surface, preferably the floor.
3. Strike the sternum (the breast bone, in the mid-line of the chest) firmly with the flat of the hand. This may be enough to re-start the heart in some cases.

Fig. 18/2 A. Position of the hands on the sternum for external cardiac compression. B. Transverse section of the thorax

4. *Start external cardiac compression* (Fig. 18/2). Place the heel of one hand on the lower third of the sternum with the second hand on top of it. In children, light pressure with one hand is sufficient.
5. Arms straight, rock forward to bring your body-weight on to the sternum, pressing it down about 4cm (1½in), thus compressing the heart against the back wall of the chest.
6. Rock back to release the pressure and repeat the sequence 60 times a minute.
7. An assistant should give mouth-to-mouth artificial respiration at the same time. (See treatment of respiratory failure, p. 213.)
8. If the operator is alone give about 15 cardiac compressions, followed by two rapid lung inflations, and then repeat.
9. Continue the sequence until the patient is either out of danger, arrives at hospital or the patient's muscles stiffen from rigor mortis which indicates that death has occurred.

EMERGENCY KIT

This should contain the following drugs and agents, and the means to administer them quickly and efficiently. Such means will include: syringes and needles; ampoules of sterile water for injection (used to dissolve doses of dry drug powder also in sterile ampoules), and ampoule files; skin cleaning swabs in tear-open sachets.

Airways, mouth-gags, tongue forceps, swabs, adequate suction apparatus, torch or pen-light.

Oxygen: This relieves anoxia due to shock, cardiac or respiratory failure. The high pressure from the cylinder must be lessened by a reducing valve and the gas administered with a mask.

Adrenaline (1:1000 solution): This is a circulatory and cardiac stimulant given by injection. It is also used in severe drug sensitivity reaction.

Hydrocortisone sodium succinate for injection: This is used in the treatment of circulatory collapse or severe drug sensitivity reaction.

Antihistamines: These are used in the treatment of drug sensitivity reaction, e.g. penicillin sensitivity.

Glyceryl trinitrate tablets: These are used for treating angina attacks.

Chapter Nineteen

CARE AND USE OF DRUGS IN DENTISTRY

A wide range of drugs is used in the local and general treatment of dental diseases. Some are kept immediately available for use in the dental surgery, while others, for the patient's home use, are supplied by the pharmacist in accordance with the dental surgeon's prescription or written order.

The DSA must always remember that all matters concerned with drugs need great responsibility on her part because of the powerful nature of many preparations and the dangers that can occur if they are carelessly handled or inappropriately administered.

MEDICINES LEGISLATION

The sale and supply of medicinal substances are controlled by the Medicines Act 1968. The Act divides these substances into three main classes:

1. *General Sale List Medicines* (GSL). Medicinal products which can, with reasonable safety, be sold or supplied otherwise than under the supervision of a Pharmacist.

2. *Pharmacy Medicines* (P). Any medicinal product which can only be sold or supplied from a pharmacy, e.g. aspirin, paracetamol and codeine tablets. The Misuse of Drugs Act 1971 provides comprehensive control over drugs of all kinds and prohibits certain activities regarding manufacture, supply and possession of Controlled Drugs, i.e. those which are known to cause addiction or drug dependence if misused. The Misuse of Drugs Regulations 1973 defines the classes of person authorised to supply and possess controlled drugs while acting in their professional capacities and lays down conditions under which these activities may be carried out. Controlled Drugs are listed in Schedules which define the rigour of control of prescribing. For example Schedule 2 includes the main addictive drugs such as the opiates (heroin, morphine and methadone).

3. *Prescription Only Medicines* (POM). Medicinal products including

Controlled Drugs that may only be sold or supplied from pharmacies in accordance with a prescription given by a registered practitioner. (A prescription is a written order from a doctor or dentist for the supply of drugs to a patient.)

A dental surgeon may keep in stock and administer certain Controlled Drugs but only in so far as is necessary for the practice of his profession. If he does use such drugs in his practice he is required by law to keep a record of their receipt which should include:

1. The date on which the drug was received
2. The name and address of the person or firm from whom it was received
3. The amount received, and
4. The form in which it was received.

These details should be recorded in a book set aside for this purpose. It is also advisable to record the occasions on which the Controlled Drug was administered, i.e. the quantity and date. Controlled Drugs must be stored in a locked, fixed receptacle for which the practitioner alone has the key. A dental surgeon is not authorised to supply these drugs other than by direct administration to a patient receiving dental treatment. However, he may prescribe such drugs for use outside the dental surgery for 'dental treatment only'.

The Dental Practitioners' Formulary (DPF) lists all the drugs and preparations that may be prescribed under the National Health Service in Britain. Since 1984 the DPF has been published in one volume together with the *British National Formulary* (BNF) which is the handbook for medical prescribing and allows the dental surgeon to identify drugs, and their actions, that patients may already be taking for general medical treatment. It is revised twice-yearly and is distributed free to all NHS practitioners.

Regulations for the control of drugs may be modified and amended from time to time and the latest details are to be found in *Medicines and Poisons Guide* published by The Pharmaceutical Press, 1 Lambeth High Street, London SE1 7JN.

CARE OF DRUGS IN THE DENTAL SURGERY

Records
As well as the Controlled Drugs records required by law, an accurate

record of the dates and quantities of other drugs received at the practice should be maintained. This not only keeps track of the drugs, but will also be of help in re-ordering new stock by indicating the rate at which individual items are used up.

Storage and security

1. All drugs must be clearly labelled at all times and in case of doubt the unidentified drug should be destroyed.
2. All drugs should be stored in cool, dry conditions. Always check the manufacturer's advice about storage conditions and make a note on the label of the expiry date of preparations that are known to deteriorate on keeping.
3. Poisons must be clearly labelled by name, plus a cautionary label marked 'Poison' together with any warning notices, e.g. 'This substance is caustic'. Poisonous liquids should be in ribbed bottles that are recognisable by touch. Poisons should be stored in a special cupboard, drawer or even a special shelf so that they are not mistaken for non-poisonous drugs. They must not be stored near foodstuffs.
4. Controlled Drugs (see Misuse of Drugs Regulations, p. 218) must be kept under the dental surgeon's personal supervision in a fixed, locked receptacle to which he alone has the key. This category of drugs is rarely required in general practice.
5. Analgesics, sedatives, hypnotics, tranquillisers and all drugs that act on the central nervous system are capable of producing a state of drug dependence or addiction in subjects to whom they are administered repeatedly and in sufficient dose. All such drugs should be kept under lock and key to avoid unauthorised use, as should the prescription pad. Theft of drugs is a matter of serious concern, and every precaution must be taken to prevent it.
6. Certain drugs, e.g. local anaesthetic solutions, penicillin, can cause hypersensitivity in members of the dental team if they are handled carelessly, even minute amounts that are allowed to come into frequent, unnecessary contact with the skin.
7. Caustic drugs, e.g. phenol, can burn the skin if they are spilt. Containers should be handled with great care and must not be stored on high shelves where an accident could splash them into the face and eyes.

ADMINISTRATION OF DRUGS

The DSA must never give a drug to a patient, not even an aspirin, without the dental surgeon's direct instruction to do so on each occasion.

Drugs may be administered to the patient by various routes.

1. Oral. This is perhaps the commonest route. The drug is taken by mouth and absorbed from the gastro-intestinal tract, e.g. aspirin.
2. Sublingual. The drug is placed under the tongue and is absorbed through the oral mucosa, e.g. glyceryl trinitrate in an angina pectoris attack. This route is rarely used in dentistry.
3. Intramuscularly, by injection into muscle, e.g. penicillin.
4. Intravenously, by injection into a vein, e.g. anaesthetic drugs.
5. Subcutaneously, by injection just beneath the skin, e.g. local anaesthetic infiltration.
6. Inhalation, breathed in and absorbed by the lungs, e.g. inhalation anaesthesia.
7. Topically, by application to the surface of the skin or tooth, e.g. topical anaesthetic ointment.

WEIGHTS AND MEASURES

Doses of drugs are calculated and expressed by the metric system:
Weight

      1000 milligrams (mg) = 1 gram (g)
      1000 grams   = 1 kilogram (kg)

Volume

      1000 millilitres (ml) = 1 litre
      1 litre is the volume of 1 kilogram of water

The strength of a solution can be expressed as a percentage, e.g.:
1g weight or 1ml volume in 100ml water = a 1% solution
5g weight or 5ml volume in 100ml water = a 5% solution

SOME DRUGS USED IN DENTISTRY

Drugs are the substances or agents that are used in the treatment or prevention of disease and to assist the healing of wounds. They can be classified according to their action and uses.

Anaesthetics (see Chapter 12)

Analgesics

Mild analgesics (anodynes). These are drugs which relieve pain without causing loss of consciousness or sensation (feeling).

    Aspirin is used to relieve pain due to infection or injury, for headache and, because of its antipyretic (fever-reducing) action, it may be taken to alleviate the symptoms of a feverish cold. It may cause gastric irritation or bleeding if taken on an empty stomach and tablets should therefore be taken after meals, crushed or dissolved in water (soluble aspirin is available). Aspirin is not suitable for infants under one year because it can cause them to have dangerous metabolic upsets.

Paracetamol is also an analgesic antipyretic used to control mild or moderate pain, and it does not seem to cause indigestion or gastric bleeding. It is, however, more dangerous than aspirin in overdosage (as little as 20 tablets) because it can cause severe liver and kidney damage.

Dihydrocodeine (DF118) is a most potent and effective analgesic given by mouth. It may cause nausea and giddiness.

Codeine is a drug obtained from opium, but without its potent effects. It is usually taken in combination with aspirin and paracetamol in a tablet.

Strong analgesics (narcotics). These include *morphine* (an opium derivative) and *pethidine*, drugs capable of relieving pain and producing a sense of well-being (euphoria) and mental detachment which makes them potentially habit-forming drugs of dependence. They are not often used in general dental practice.

Antiseptics and disinfectants

Antiseptics are substances which inhibit or arrest the growth and multiplication of bacteria. *Disinfectants* destroy bacteria but cannot be relied upon to kill spores and viruses (see Chapter 5). 'Germicides' kill 'germs'. Most antiseptics may be applied to living tissues without causing injury, but disinfectants is the term usually applied to agents destroying pathogenic organisms and used for large-scale disinfection of inanimate objects.

1. **Physical:** Instruments and utensils may be disinfected by boiling them in water (100°C) for 15 minutes.

2. **Alcohol:** A 60–95% solution is rapidly bactericidal and a 70% solution is an antiseptic used for storing sterile instruments for very short periods and also for cleaning skin or working surfaces in the surgery.

3. **Aldehydes:**

Formaldehyde (as formalin solution) is a strong disinfectant that is irritant to the skin. A 2% solution is germicidal after 30 minutes and a 4–8% solution may kill spores after 24 hours. Formaldehyde vapour has a very slow sterilising action.

Glutaraldehyde is an alkaline solution which is claimed to be a rapid sporicide (i.e. it kills organisms and their spores) and is suitable for surface sterilisation. Hard surfaced, non-absorbent instruments should be totally immersed in a 2% activated solution for three hours (8 to 10 is safer). All the solution must be washed off with sterile water.

Paraformaldehyde, a solid polymer which slowly releases formalin at body temperature, is a tissue-fixing agent used in pulp mummification.

4. **Dyes:** Solutions of certain dyes act as mild antibacterial agents, e.g. crystal violet, brilliant green. They are rarely used in dentistry.

5. **Halogens:**

Iodine: A dilute solution may sometimes be used as an antiseptic and its stain indicates the area of application.

Iodoform, occurs as yellow crystals, which slowly liberate iodine. It is used as an antiseptic agent to treat infected wounds and in certain root canal therapy agents. BIPP (bismuth, iodoform and paraffin paste) is an ointment used on ribbon gauze to dress extraction sockets.

Chlorine: 1% sodium hypochlorite solution (Milton) is a non-toxic antiseptic and germicide. It may be used to irrigate root canals. Dilute solutions are used to disinfect surfaces and equipment. Stronger solutions of the hypochlorite are caustic and also act as bleaching solutions.

6. **Oxidising agents:** *Hydrogen peroxide* has antiseptic, deodorant and bleaching properties. It is regarded as a weak germicide of short duration. A 20 volume solution, diluted 1:20 with water, is used as a mouthwash and as a debris-removing agent in root canal therapy. ('20 volume' means that 20 volumes of oxygen can be released from 1 volume of the solution.)

7. **Phenols and cresols:**

Phenol (carbolic acid) is a strong disinfectant and protoplasmic poison. Pure phenol and strong solutions are caustic and can rapidly penetrate and kill skin and mucous membranes. The local antidote is to wash the affected body surface with alcohol and apply glycerin to the burn.

A 1% phenol solution is a disinfectant but is rarely used on the tissues because of the danger of absorption into the body.

A 5% phenol solution is a disinfectant but cannot be relied upon to kill spores.

Carbolised resin is used to devitalise the dental pulp.

Monochlorophenol with *camphor* is used as a root canal disinfectant.

Cresol (tricresol) is a disinfectant used in root canal therapy.

Thymol is a phenolic disinfectant used in mouthwashes.

Hexachlorophane: Soaps and creams containing 1 to 3 per cent are used to reduce the bacterial flora on the skin. It should not be applied repeatedly to the whole surface of the body. (Particularly in infants.)

Creosote is derived from tar. It acts as a mild local analgesic and antiseptic and is used in pulp therapy and root canal treatment.

Eugenol is the essential constituent of clove oil (clove oil contains 85 to 90 per cent of eugenol). It has an antiseptic and obtundent action and is used with zinc oxide powder as a basis of many temporary filling materials and gingival packs. It may be used as an antiseptic in pulp and root canal therapy.

8. **Surface active agents:**

Benzalkonium chloride (Zephiran (USA), Roccal) is a quaternary

222

ammonium compound and forms non-irritant, detergent, antiseptic and disinfectant solutions. A 0.1% solution can be used for pre-operative cleaning and disinfection of the skin and, with the addition of rust-inhibitors (sodium nitrite and sodium carbonate) for the short-term storage of sterile instruments.

Cetrimide (Cetavlon): A 0.5% in 70% alcohol solution is used for pre-operative disinfection of the skin. An aqueous solution of 1% can be used for cleaning utensils.

9. Chlorhexidine agents:

Chlorhexidine (Hibitane) as a 1% solution can be used for pre-operative disinfection of the skin. Dilute solutions can be used as a mouth wash.

Antibiotics

These are drugs, themselves derived from living organisms or moulds, which are capable of killing or inhibiting the growth of certain bacteria in the body. They are of great value in the treatment of severe infections in conjunction with standard surgical methods, e.g. the drainage of abscesses. In certain conditions, e.g. the presence of heart valve lesions after rheumatic fever, they may be given to prevent postoperative infective complications. Sensitisation to certain antibiotics, especially penicillin, can occur both to patients under treatment and to anyone else handling the drug without proper care. Such sensitivity can cause skin rashes and bronchial spasm upon further exposure to the drug and these unpleasant and even dangerous effects have to be treated with antihistamine drugs or adrenaline injections.

Penicillin is the most effective antibiotic. It may be administered by injection intramuscularly or by buffered oral preparations. No patient must be given penicillin without first asking them if they have any previous history of sensitivity to the drug. Ampicillin and amoxycillin are semi-synthetic penicillins.

Tetracycline is usually given orally for general infections. Tetracycline mouth-baths are used for primary herpetic stomatitis. If this drug is taken during the period of tooth mineralisation it may be deposited in the calcifying areas and cause discolouration.

Erythromycin is sometimes used to treat infections in patients who are sensitive to penicillin.
(See Fungicides.)

Antihistamines

These are drugs used in the treatment of skin rashes and other reactions caused by sensitivity to certain substances, e.g. penicillin. They include *chlorpheniramine maleate* (Piriton) and *promethazine hydrochloride*

(Phenergan). These drugs themselves may have side-effects causing dry mouth and drowsiness.

Caustics

These are substances that cause local burns or tissue death.

They include *trichloroacetic acid* (used for rapid removal of mucous membrane), *phenol, solid silver nitrate*.

Corticosteroids

These are products of the adrenal cortex (a ductless gland). Their action is to modify tissue reactions to injury and inflammation by suppressing the disease function and they have an effect on the general circulation and blood pressure. They are used topically in the form of *hydrocortisone sodium succinate* lozenges (Corlan Pellets) and creams, *triamcinolone acetonide* paste (Adcortyl-A in Orabase), in the treatment of aphthous ulceration of the mouth.

Patients under medical treatment with steroids for general diseases such as arthritis and chronic skin diseases are likely to suffer severe shock and collapse during routine anaesthesia and surgery unless they are protected by an increased pre-operative dose of the drug given in direct consultation with their medical adviser. Hydrocortisone sodium succinate injection is used to treat the sudden onset of anaphylactic shock and circulatory collapse (see Chapter 18).

Fungicides

These kill fungi and moulds; *fungistats* inhibit their growth. They are used in the treatment of thrush, 'denture sore mouth', and occasionally in root canal therapy.

Nystatin is used topically in the form of tablets which are allowed to dissolve in the mouth.

Amphotericin B (Fungilin) is used in the same way but has a less unpleasant taste.

Sodium caprylate solution is used in root canal therapy.

Haemostatics

These are drugs and measures which arrest bleeding.
1. *Physical measures to be taken are:* pressure, pack, suture, absorbable haemostatics.
   Absorbable haemostatics: Oxidised cellulose gauze is used dry in the wound and, with the escaping blood, forms an artificial clot. So does calcium alginate and absorbable gelatin sponge.
2. *Vasoconstrictors:* The topical application of adrenaline solution causes

constriction of the capillaries and reduces local bleeding.

3. *Haemostatic sera:* Russell's viper venom (Stypven) is applied to the wound on wool or is dropped from a needle (*never* injected) and causes rapid coagulation of blood.

Hypnotics

These are drugs which induce sleep.

Nitrazepam may be given the night before a dental operation to ensure a good night's sleep. The after-effects include delayed reaction times the next day.

Chloral hydrate is often used for children and lasts about eight hours. Triclofos is similar to chloral hydrate but is less irritant to the stomach and can be given in tablet or syrup form.

(See Sedatives.)

Medical gas cylinders

Labelling and identification colours for medical gas cylinders, British Standard, 1955.

Gas	Symbol	Colour of cylinder	Colour of valve end of cylinder
Oxygen	O_2	Black	White
Nitrous oxide	N_2O	Blue	–
Air (compressed) airotors, laboratory uses, etc	–	French grey	White and black

The name of the gas is stencilled on the body of each cylinder and is also clearly stamped on the metal cylinder valve.

Mummifying agents

These kill tissues and render them resistant to subsequent growth of organisms. They are used in certain forms of pulp therapy, especially in deciduous teeth. They include *formaldehyde, para-formaldehyde, iodoform* and *cresol*.

Obtundents

These are drugs used locally to dull the sensitivity of dentine during excavation of a cavity. They include *eugenol, phenol* and *cresol*.

Sedatives and tranquillisers

Sedatives depress the central nervous system, have a mood calming effect and soothe the anxious patient. They also dull the faculties and make the patient sleepy so that he is unable to carry out his normal activity. They reduce pre-operative apprehension if given an hour or so beforehand.

Diazepam (Valium) and *chloral hydrate* act as sedatives in sub-hypnotic doses (see Hypnotics).

Tranquillisers give the patient 'peace of mind'. They have a calming effect without impairing the patient's alertness. They are often taken for long periods, under careful medical supervision. Their effectiveness varies widely in different patients. *Chlordiazepoxide* (Librium) and *diazepam* (Valium) are used as tranquillisers.

Note: Patients taking these drugs must not attempt to drive a car or work machinery. They must not take alcohol, which potentiates the action of the drug.

Emergency kit (see Chapter 18, page 216)

Chapter Twenty

STUDY METHODS AND
EXAMINATION TECHNIQUE

It is always easier to settle down to the continuous attainment of knowledge over a prolonged period if this is being done to achieve some specific end. From the outset a constantly growing and expanding knowledge of dentistry will make your everyday work far more interesting and worthwhile, but if you are also preparing to take a recognised professional examination for Dental Surgery Assistants you know that every moment of study is taking you nearer to a most important personal achievement. To have gained a qualification of this sort brings considerable satisfaction and self-confidence and will give you status in personal advancement and future job applications.

Anyone who has the normal curiosity and interest about their work is capable of getting down to study and, if you go about it in an organised and planned way, there is a great deal of enjoyment to be gained from the sense of purpose that is quickly felt. Planned study can be carried out with an increasing economy of effort as your mind becomes accustomed to the habits of observing, remembering and thinking to some definite purpose.

Before setting out on a course of study you are recommended to discuss the matter with your own dental surgeon. You can also obtain valuable advice by writing to your national examining board for details of their examination, their syllabus of study and copies of recent examination papers. You should also contact local colleges or dental schools for particulars of their DSA courses.

Theoretical and practical tuition
Several methods of tuition are available:
1. Full-time courses at dental schools or day colleges
2. Part-time evening or other classes at colleges
3. Private coaching
4. Correspondence courses
5. Self-tuition.

As well as theoretical knowledge the trained DSA must also have a

227

considerable amount of practical chairside experience that can only be gained in the dental surgery assisting the dental surgeon – who is thus the most important teacher you will have.

Most people find it stimulating to attend a regular course of lectures and classes. There is help, encouragement and enthusiasm from the teacher and a chance to measure your own standards against those of the other students. However, your teacher cannot learn the facts for you and the main effort of study still lies in organised, planned self-tuition, day by day.

STUDY METHODS

From the start allocate a certain amount of time each day for study and make sure that you keep to it rigidly. It is important not to be too ambitious about this time allocation. One hour a day at first will be ample. Small amounts of work, regularly carried out, will achieve a great effect. Try to choose a time of day when you will be feeling fresh and alert. You will soon get into the study habit.

Make out two timetables, one the long-term strategical plan of work which will divide up the total course, and the other a short-term tactical timetable for the next week or so. The latter means that you will soon feel the stimulating satisfaction, gained by achieving working targets and deadlines, that is so important in maintaining a long-term planned effort. In the long-term timetable make sure that you leave some margin of time for unpredictable events such as holidays, illness and so on. Make sure that you have some completely free time in your timetable for rest and recreation. When you reach the point of being able to study for more than an hour at a time, take five minutes' rest away from your work every hour; even this short break will refresh your mind considerably.

Try to find the best place and conditions for your study periods. The things that you *must* have are a desk or a table, a comfortable chair (but not too comfortable!), adequate light, heating and ventilation in a room that is reasonably quiet. Keep your books and study things together so that you can start each period of study without having the delay or distraction of time-wasting preparation. Tell your family and friends that you are studying and the hours that you have set aside for it. This will strengthen your resolve to get down to work (you won't want to let yourself down!) and also stop them from unwittingly interrupting your new work habits.

Remember that there are many odd moments during the day that can also be used for study and revision. For example, the time spent in public transport on the journey to and from work and spare minutes during the lunch break, can be used to your advantage if you always carry a book, journal or notes about with you.

Notebooks

It is important to keep clear and accurate written notes of your studies, limiting them to essential facts and principles. This will give the immediate benefit of a sense of progress and achievement; it will practise the important arts of understanding and organising facts and writing them down; it will improve your spelling and handwriting and, most valuable of all, you will be assembling your notes for pre-examination revision. These notes are best kept in a loose-leaf file.

A second pocket notebook can be carried at all times so that you can make an immediate note of items that you come across during the working day that are worthy of adding to your best loose-leaf file later on. Lecture notes may also be taken down quickly in a rough book and then copied out carefully into the file as soon as possible for this is a very effective method of early revision. Watch out for the correct spelling of unfamiliar words heard in lectures.

Reading

Reading forms an important part of your studies and you should develop a new technique if you are to get the most help possible from a book. First of all do not be daunted by the length of it or try to get through a certain number of pages each day. Start by skimming through the whole book trying to see the shape of it all, how the chapters are laid out and the broad outline of what its author is trying to convey to you. Then go back to the beginning and read it in detail at the rate you find most suitable, making notes or underlining key words and sentences. Parts of it will seem more difficult and will need more time, others will go quickly. Finally, read the whole thing through again in the light of your own growing personal knowledge and experience. All the time try to carry any new facts into the dental surgery with you to test and perhaps relate them to your everyday practical work. Get your dental surgeon to discuss them with you – most dentists love to talk about their work to an intelligent and enquiring audience!

Borrow dental journals and keep an eye on current trends and materials. In free moments talk to the dental technician, the oral hygienist, the anaesthetist, the other dental surgery assistants and the dental company representatives about dentistry for they are all valuable sources of information. Very few people will resent such curiosity and most will be flattered that you have asked them.

Revision

General revision should be carried out currently during the whole period of study and not left entirely until the last week or two before the examination.

Make sure that your timetable allows you to go back and read through your notes at frequent intervals. Diligent, methodical work will mean that little intensive revision is required and will play its part in reducing pre-examination tensions. You should test yourself frequently from the outset of your studies to make sure that you can remember important lists of facts. This is best done by actively reciting them from memory or writing them down, rather than passively reading them through. Make up mnemonics to help you to recall long lists of facts by constructing a sentence or word using the initial letters of the facts in question (e.g. the branches of the external carotid artery:Superior thyroid, Lingual, Facial, Occipital, ascending Pharyngeal, posterior Auricular, Superficial temporal and Maxillary can be recalled from the mnemonic 'Some Little Fellows Open Purses And Steal Money').

Self-testing can be extended by working through questions from old examination papers. This will help you to gain further practice in expressing yourself in writing and will train you up to the standard of being able to write for a prolonged period in the actual examination.

Pre-examination

Try to spend a restful day before the actual examination, though some people feel happier just glancing through their notebooks again. Get together all the things that you will need in the examination and work out the route to the examination hall. Go to bed early and try to put the affairs of the next day out of your mind.

EXAMINATION

On the morning of the examination get up early and have a good breakfast. Some people feel hungry during a three-hour examination once the first excitement has worn off, so if you do not normally eat a large breakfast, take a few glucose sweets in your pocket. During the written examination they will pacify the pangs of hunger and raise your blood sugar when you most need it. This must be the only occasion when a dental surgeon will advocate sweets between meals!

You will have collected together your 'Examination Kit':

A clean uniform and cap (plain shoes, no jewellery, neat hair style, clean fingernails, no vail varnish, discreet make-up and perfume) which will be worn for the practical and oral examination. Facilities for changing will be available at the examination centre.

Admission card

Fountain pen and refill, or ball-point pens

Pencils and sharpener   Coloured pencils

Rubber   Ruler   Watch

Arrive at the examination hall early. This will allow you to get settled and used to the surroundings. Remember that nervousness before an examination is universal. Some of the candidates like to 'unload' their tensions onto others, so be careful who you chum up with in the moments before the examination room doors are opened to you. Your own slight tension is good for you, although you may find it hard to believe. The stressed feeling can be used to give you that special elation that means that you will be able to do your best. Make that energy work for you by keeping cool and collected. Nervousness on its own will not fail an examination, but bland over-confidence can do so.

Once in the examination room, settle down and take your time to read the paper through, taking particular care to read the examiner's instructions at the top of the page. Is the timing and the number of questions to be answered the same as in the previous papers you have practised on? Plan out how long you have to answer each question. Choose which essay questions you are going to answer and read them through again checking for the key words that precisely define the extent of the answer required. Jot down an outline of your answers – just main paragraph headings and fact lists. As you do this you will find that your previously despised tension will have your mind working faster than you thought possible and ideas and facts will come rushing from your memory just as you need them.

Now you can start to write out your answers. Start off with the easiest question first, keep your answer simple and with the examiner in mind as if you were explaining it all to him. Get the points in order and make headings. Put in some simple drawings if they are appropriate and label them carefully. Try to set the whole thing out in a neat, attractive and legible style. It may be 'window-dressing' but examiners are human beings! Watch the time constantly for you must answer all the questions if you are to get good marks. If time presses before you can complete the answer to the last question at least jot down the headings for they can gain precious marks for you. The examiner is not trying to fail you so give him all the help you possibly can! Finally, read through your answers carefully. You'll be surprised at the number of punctuation and spelling mistakes you will have made.

In some cases part of the written examination is in the form of *multiple choice questions*. A printed questionnaire is provided which has spaces for the candidate to say which of the two or three alternative answers provided is correct or else to write in one- or two-word answers. This is a pure test of knowledge and overcomes the difficulty that some people have in expressing themselves in essay questions. Work your way through the questions and if any of them hold you up leave them, complete all the easy questions first and then go back to the one or two that you find difficult. In this way you will not miss any opportunity to gain marks. There may also be short answer questions and a charting test, as well as the essay type question in the second part of the written paper.

Between the paper and the practical and oral examination, if they are all on the same day, try to have a light, quiet meal and, if possible, a short walk in the fresh air.

In the oral and practical parts of the examination you will be given 'spotter' tests, practical tests and an oral examination. The 'spotter' test will ask you to identify and list by name and usage groups of dental instruments and materials. In the practical test you will be asked to carry out a specific technique, such as mixing an impression material and loading a tray, or mounting radiographs on a hanger. In the oral examination the examiner will spend a short time asking questions about all aspects of dentistry, both practical and theoretical.

In all this you must be aware constantly of the impression you are trying to make. This will be reflected in your dress, your posture, your manner and your voice. Remember to speak up always and even smile occasionally.

For further details, the intending student should consult the syllabus and regulations for the appropriate National Certificate of the Examining Board for Dental Surgery Assistants. This will include up-to-date details of the requirements for eligibility for entrance to the examination and information of what the examination includes. Copies of past examination papers are also available. In Britain such details for this national examination may be obtained from: The Association of Dental Surgery Assistants, DSA House, 29 London Street, Fleetwood, Lancashire FY7 6JY.

When you have passed the examination, do not be tempted to allow your study habit and knowledge to be neglected. Dentistry is constantly expanding. The trained Dental Surgery Assistant owes it to herself and her profession to keep alert and up-to-date.

Chapter Twenty-One

EXAMINATION QUESTIONS

The following represent a selection of the questions set in recent examination papers by the Examining Board for Dental Surgery Assistants for the National Certificate. They are reproduced by permission of the Board.

1. (a) Draw a labelled diagram illustrating the blood circulation in the body and show the routes taken by oxygenated and deoxygenated blood.
    (b) What is the composition of blood?
    (c) Define the term 'haemorrhage'.
2. (a) Name the salivary glands and describe their location.
    (b) What are the functions of saliva?
    (c) Why is it necessary to eliminate saliva during certain clinical procedures and what methods are used?
3. Describe the muscles of mastication and their attachments.
4. What is the nerve supply of the teeth and gums of the upper jaw? A dental surgeon is to give an injection of local anaesthetic for a procedure on an upper tooth. What preparations would you make?
5. Write notes on the care, maintenance and sterilisation of dental handpieces.
6. What is the significance of the following with regard to dental treatment:
    (a) pregnancy
    (b) serum hepatitis
    (c) rheumatic fever
7. Briefly explain what is meant by Angle's Classification. Describe the methods which may be used to correct malocclusion. Outline what oral hygiene regime would be advised during treatment and say what instructions you would give with regard to the care of the appliance.
8. Describe the dangers of working with:
    (a) x-rays
    (b) mercury
    What precautions should the dental surgery assistant take to protect herself and the patient?

9. Write notes on each of the following:
    (a) plaque
    (b) calculus
    (c) interdental cleaning
    (d) disclosing agents
10. How would you prepare the surgery at the start of the day?
11. How can a dental surgery assistant help the dental surgeon with a patient before, during, and after a general anaesthetic?
    What instructions should be given to a patient before and after a general anaesthetic?
    How should a patient be prepared for the operation on attendance?
12. List the materials and instruments which may be required during the restoration with amalgam of a badly broken down lower molar. Describe how you would assist the dentist during this procedure.
13. Why may teeth require crowning?
    Describe the stages in crowning a root-filled upper anterior tooth.
    List the various materials and instruments used and describe the part played by the DSA at each stage.
14. What is an immediate denture? Describe the various stages in its construction and detail the preparations to be made by the DSA for the visit when the denture will be inserted.
15. What are the main types of impression materials? Give the principal uses of each.
16. How can fluoride help dental health? Describe how it may be used:
    (a) by a patient at home
    (b) by the dentist
    (c) by the community as a whole
17. (a) What measures should be adopted by a girl aged 12 to ensure good dental health?
    (b) How would you convince her of the importance of oral health?
18. Describe the role of the DSA in each of the following emergencies if they occur in the dental surgery:
    (a) epileptic fit
    (b) fainting attack
    (c) cardiac arrest
    (d) vomiting associated with general anaesthesia
19. What are the main dental diseases and how may they be prevented or minimised?
    (a) by the local authority
    (b) by the dentist
    (c) by the dental surgery assistant
    (d) by the patient

20. Write short notes on the following giving their uses in dentistry:
    (a) halothane (Fluothane)
    (b) antibiotics
    (c) analgesics
    (d) adrenalin

'Spotter' tests

The following four pictures (pages 236–9) show the trolley setting for various procedures. The instruments are not named, but all will be found in the text. You can use them to test your knowledge.

Fig. 21/1 Basic conservation tray

Fig. 21/2 Basic scale and polish tray

Fig. 21/3 Basic rubber dam application tray

Fig. 21/4 Basic oral surgery trolley set up

Further Reading

Combe, E. C. (1977). *Notes on Dental Materials*, 3rd edition. Churchill Livingstone, Edinburgh.

Dental Practitioner's Formulary (1983). British Medical Association, London.

Downer, G. C. (1975). *Dental Morphology – an illustrated guide*. John Wright and Sons Limited, Bristol.

Erridge, P. L. (1979). *Self-assessment Questions and Answers for Dental Assistants*. John Wright and Sons Limited, Bristol.

Forrest, J. O. (1981). *Preventive Dentistry*, 2nd edition. John Wright and Sons Limited, Bristol.

Frommer, H. H. (1978). *Radiology for Dental Auxiliaries*, 2nd edition. C. V. Mosby Co, St Louis.

Gelbier, S. and Copley, M. A. H. (1977). *Handbook for Dental Surgery Assistants and Other Ancillary Workers*, 2nd edition. John Wright and Sons Limited, Bristol.

Gray's Anatomy, 36th edition (1981). Longman Group Limited, Edinburgh. (The sections relating to the teeth and jaws.)

Heinemann Modern Dictionary for Dental Students, 2nd edition (1973). William Heinemann Medical Books Limited, London.

Levison, H. (1978). *Textbook for Dental Nurses*, 5th edition. Blackwell Scientific Publications Limited, Oxford.

Moore, J. R. and Gillbe, G. V. (1976). *Principals of Oral Surgery*, 2nd edition. Manchester University Press, Manchester.

Pearce, E. (1975). *Anatomy and Physiology for Nurses*, 16th edition. Faber and Faber, London.

Renson, C. E. (ed) (1978). *Oral Disease*. Update Publications, London.

Smith, N. J. D. (1980). *Dental Radiography*. Blackwell Scientific Publications Limited, Oxford.

How to Study by Harry Maddox. Pan Books, London.

Radiological Protection in Dental Practice★
Emergencies in Dental Practice★

★These two pamphlets are published by the Department of Health and Social Security, London SE1 6BY

Notes for Students of Dental Health Education – Health Education Council Publication.

Index

NOTES

NOTES

NOTES

NOTES